ECMO: A Practical Guide to Management

Ahmed Reda Taha • Mark Caridi-Scheible
Eric R. Leiendecker • Casey Frost Miller
Editors

ECMO: A Practical Guide to Management

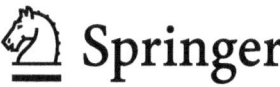 Springer

Editors
Ahmed Reda Taha
Cleveland Clinic
Critical Care Institute
Abu Dhabi, United Arab Emirates

Eric R. Leiendecker
Emory University Hospital
Atlanta, GA, USA

Mark Caridi-Scheible
Emory University Hospital
Atlanta, GA, USA

Casey Frost Miller
Department of Cardiothoracic Surgery
Emory University Hospital
Atlanta, GA, USA

ISBN 978-3-031-59633-9   ISBN 978-3-031-59634-6   (eBook)
https://doi.org/10.1007/978-3-031-59634-6

This Springer imprint is published by the registered company Springer Nature Switzerland AG
The registered company address is: Gewerbestrasse 11, 6330 Cham, Switzerland

If disposing of this product, please recycle the paper.

Preface

In recent years, extracorporeal membrane oxygenation (ECMO) has advanced rapidly in its prevalence and ease of use. In our opinion, it is rapidly becoming the standard of care for the management of severe acute respiratory distress syndrome (ARDS). However, its adoption has been limited outside of relatively few large hospitals in primarily very wealthy nations. Although in part improving as the cost of the equipment and associated resources declines, a significant barrier to its use remains in the expertise required to manage the patient. There are many reasons for this limited expertise, but one is lack of access to training opportunities and educational materials. There are only a few existing reference books, but they are often too expensive for the average practitioner or hospital system to use as general reference material for training. Cheaper volumes tend to be too basic or of low quality. We sought to remedy this situation with a high-quality but open-access textbook.

This textbook is meant to be a practical guide to the management of ECMO by the entire ECMO team from specialists to physicians. It discusses the core physiological principles necessary to the understanding of its management but then also describes how to practically apply these principles on a day-to-day basis. It is meant to be focused and concise, with an emphasis on translating theory to actual application on equipment and patients.

We hope that its primary use will be as a didactic tool for ECMO programs to provide training to both their new and continuing learners. In general, it will be targeted toward bedside providers (physicians, mid-level providers, perfusionists); however, it will still be a useful reference material for nurses, respiratory therapists, and others on the team.

This book should not be seen as definitive, but rather as a good place to start your ECMO journey. The authors encourage the reader to continue to learn from multiple sources, and especially to become familiar with guidelines and recommendations from the Extracorporeal Life Support Organization (ELSO, elso.org). It should be noted that while we are strong advocates of ELSO, we do not speak for the organization and are not endorsed by them.

The authors who wrote this book are themselves experienced practitioners of ECMO and have a passion for education both at their home institutions and through academic work nationally and internationally. We hope that you become as ardent supporters of ECMO as we have and that you eventually want to give back to the ECMO community as a whole.

We thank you sincerely for your readership and support.

Atlanta, GA, USA   Mark Caridi-Scheible
Abu Dhabi, United Arab Emirates   Ahmed Reda Taha

Contents

Chapter 1
History of ECMO

Eric R. Leiendecker

Development of Extracorporeal Support

The story of extracorporeal support is one of identifying a physiologic problem and using human ingenuity to advance a technology to bypass that problem. Many people attribute this to Dr. Gibbon's fateful encounter with a patient with a pulmonary embolism in 1931 during his training at Harvard Medical School. It was here he so famously remarked, "During that long night, helplessly watching the patient struggle for life as her blood became darker … the idea naturally occurred to me that if it were possible to remove continuously some of the blue blood … put oxygen into that blood … and then to inject continuously the now-red blood back into the patient's arteries, we might have saved her life" [1]. This impotent experience coincided with the growing desire to expand the practice of cardiac surgery that had seen slow growth through the postwar 1940s and was largely limited by the need for a cardiopulmonary bypass machine in order to address congenital and valvular heart disease. Up until this point, the practice had been restricted to operations done without the need for mechanical support, such as Blalock-Taussig shunts and aortic coarctation repair. These two ambitions came together to drive the development of a support modality, which continues to grow in utility and importance. Prior to this intersection, there had been academic interest in extracorporeal support.

In order to achieve extracorporeal support, two problems were needing to be solved. First, there was the question of oxygenation and how to achieve this without the lungs. Second and somewhat easier to navigate was the problem of blood flow and how to provide the requisite cardiac replacement. As far back as the mid-1600s, Dr. Robert Hooke had been able to demonstrate that inflation and deflation of the lungs were not necessary for the blood in order for gas exchange to occur.

E. R. Leiendecker (✉)
Emory University Hospital, Atlanta, GA, USA
e-mail: eric.richard.leiendecker@emory.edu

© The Author(s), under exclusive license to Springer Nature Switzerland AG 2024
A. R. Taha et al. (eds.), *ECMO: A Practical Guide to Management*,
https://doi.org/10.1007/978-3-031-59634-6_1

Beyond this, he speculated that simply exposing the blood to the air may be sufficient for the gas exchange to occur, meaning the presence of the lungs is not essential. With this simple statement, Dr. Hooke summarized what would become the crucial consideration in the development of extracorporeal support: How do we achieve gas exchange and do the work of the lungs in the case where the patient's lungs cannot? Expanding on Hooke's work and postulation that direct contact with air may suffice, physicians in the mid-1800s showed that shaking together blood and air in a balloon would lead to gas transfer, a demonstration which paved the way for the development of the first modern extracorporeal oxygenator—the bubble oxygenator, developed in Germany in 1882 and used to perfuse a dissected kidney. This oxygenator, a rudimentary design, used air introduced into a venous reservoir to increase the ambient pressure and then force now oxygenated blood into a second arterial reservoir from which they used the blood to perfuse the organ. This design would later be greatly improved upon by Clark, Gollan, and Gupta in the early 1950s when they described their use of an all-glass bubble oxygenator [2].

It was the screen oxygenator though that reigned superior and was begun to be used in humans. Bjork (famous for the development of the Bjork-Shiley mechanical valve) first described this technology in 1948 and its use in providing oxygenated blood to a dog [3]. However, it was Dr. Gibbon's vision that finally came to fruition in 1953 with his first use of an oxygenator to facilitate cardiac surgery, in this case the attempted closure of an atrial septal defect (though this patient did not survive and was found not to have an ASD but instead a patent ductus arteriosus). The membrane he used consisted of six to eight wire mesh screens standing vertical and in parallel encased in a plastic housing. Venous blood flowed down these screens forming a thin layer of blood and allowing for gas exchange while exposed to a flow of oxygen over the surface of the screens [4]. Of course, others were working in parallel with Dr. Gibbon to develop a heart-lung machine to achieve the extracorporeal support needed to drive the field of cardiac surgery forward. One of the more macabre examples of this being Dr. William Mustard in Toronto, originally an orthopedic surgeon, who developed a heart machine using isolated monkey lungs as the oxygenator. In this case, the blood goes from the patient's cavae/atria through a venous reservoir and through the PA of a pair of monkey lungs, through these lungs and to an arterial reservoir and back to the patient. The lungs were manually ventilated by instilling 100% oxygen via a tube in the trachea, and a relief valve was opened in a rhythmic fashion [5]. For obvious reasons, this model of oxygenation was short lived, and attention narrowed on the use of screens or films (Fig. 1.1: Dr. Mustard's machine utilizing rhesus monkey lungs).

A natural extension of the screen oxygenators became the disc oxygenator for which Kay and Cross out of Cleveland, Ohio, gained recognition. Their oxygenator used a series of corrugated flat discs on a central drive shaft spinning at 120 revolutions per minute with venous blood on them; this spinning created a thin layer of blood, which would then be oxygenated by the high partial pressure in the oxygen-rich environment within the tube where this driveshaft was housed. While this form of oxygenator dominated the field up until the 1970s, it was not without issue. In

Fig. 1.1 Dr. Mustard's heart-lung machine using rhesus monkey lungs (1957)

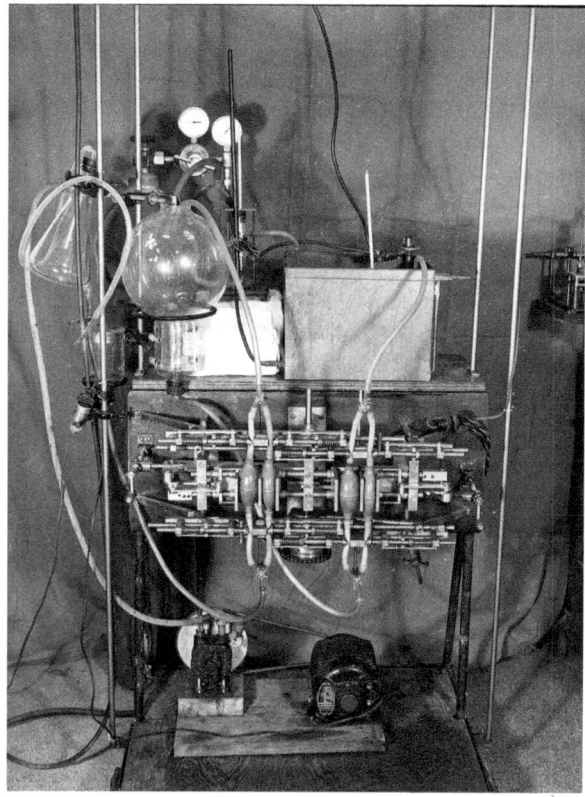

Fig. 1.2 Kay-Cross rotating disc oxygenator (1951)

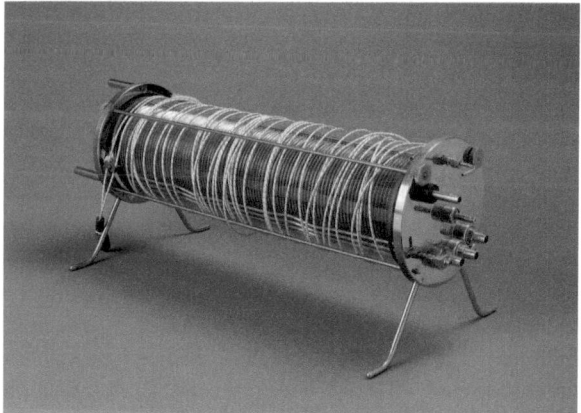

order to conserve blood, there was a need to make the housing as compact as possible, which meant the space between the discs and the housing was narrow and facilitated foaming and led to RBC destruction and sheering of clotting factors as the disc spun [6] (Fig. 1.2: Kay-Cross rotating disc oxygenator).

That is, until Jay McLean demonstrated that a substance isolated from dog organs would prevent coagulation, this substance came to be known as heparin and is the one we are surely all familiar with [7]. This solving of the coagulation issue opened up the possibility of whole-body perfusion and the development of the modern concept of extracorporeal support. However, it would be some time before the use of protamine to reverse heparin would be described and eventually replace the use of the nephrotoxic hexadimethrine bromide, another cationic agent that binds heparin [8].

Bubble oxygenators, as well, would continue to evolve following their description in 1950 by Clarke, Gollan, and Gupta. Through their work, it was found that the size of the bubbles and the rate of gas flow mattered for differing reasons [9]. Smaller bubbles resulted in larger surface area-to-volume ratios, which increased the rate of oxygen uptake, though these smaller bubbles were also less buoyant and remained in solution leading to increased rates of air emboli. From this, they were able to remark on the optimal bubble size and utility of a heterogeneous mixture of various sized bubbles for effecting oxygen transfer. In regard to CO_2 elimination, this group was able to illustrate that this occurs by diffusion. The implication of this being the gas vented from the oxygenator cannot have a high partial pressure of CO_2 than the blood, or diffusion would not occur. Thus, the elimination of CO_2 is dependent on the partial pressure gradient from blood to air, and this gradient can be kept high by increasing the rate of gas flow through the oxygenator. This is analogous to the modern-day equivalent of "sweep gas" flow rates. In the DeWall bubble oxygenator that typified this technology, oxygen was bubbled through the blood in a vertical oxygenating chamber. This would create a layer of foamy blood that would go from the oxygenating chamber to the defoaming chamber where silicone lining decreased the surface tension of the smaller bubbles forcing them to combine into larger bubbles, which would leave the blood vertically while the blood would be pumped downwards. This simple design allowed reliable gas exchange, and the lack of moving parts or mechanical aspects made this an appealing option in a time of numerous types of oxygenators being developed. Dr. Lillehei started using these in his work in 1955, and following this, the DeWall bubble oxygenator became the dominant oxygenator used until the 1970s [10].

At the same time as others were working on artificial oxygenators, Dr. Lillehei and his colleagues were engaging in preclinical work using cross circulation. Reportedly, one of his colleagues' wife was pregnant, which spurred the conversation regarding the use of one circulation to support two bodies. After creating an animal model that showed good outcomes, it was time to adapt this technology to humans. In 1954, Lillehei and his colleagues took a 3-year-old patient to the OR for correction of a VSD and used the patient's father as the extracorporeal oxygenator by removing blood from the patient's vena cava and returning it through a cannula in the father's femoral vein. This blood then was oxygenated prior to being shunted from the father's femoral artery and into the ascending aorta of the patient for total-body perfusion [11]. While initial reaction to news of this breakthrough was tepid given the chance of a 200% mortality, the Minnesota group published a case series of 45 patients in which this modality was used, followed by a 30-year follow-up of

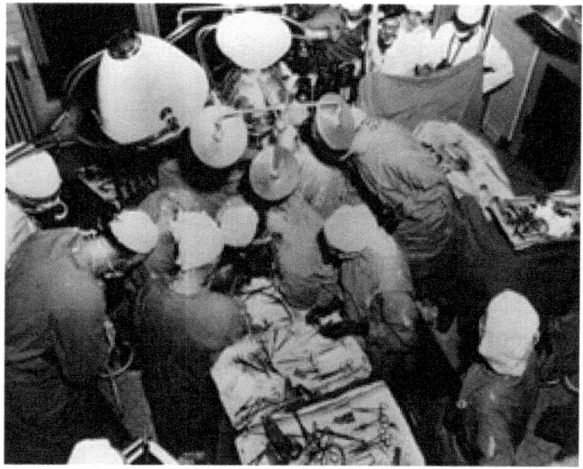

Fig. 1.3 Dr. Lillehei utilizing cross circulation to perform a VSD closure (1954)

survivors. While all 45 of the donors survived, only 20 of the patients survived to be termed "long-term" [12] (Fig. 1.3: Dr. Lillehei utilizing cross circulation in his first case).

These oxygenators, would of course, have to be attached to some sort of machine to replace the work done by the heart and lungs. In Detroit, engineers from General Motors were recruited by Forest Dodrill to create a heart pump. Their device, resembling a Cadillac V-12 engine, was composed of six cylinders made of steel, glass, and rubber, which in turn used air pressure and vacuum pumps to circulate blood. He had initially planned to use this machine for right or left heart bypass for simpler operations, and in 1952, this machine was used for 50 min to allow a mitral valve procedure on a 41-year-old man [13]. Simultaneously, John Gibbon, in Philadelphia, was attaching his screen oxygenator to a machine driven by DeBakey roller clamps, using assistance from IBM in the form of engineers, that he used in 1953 for his ASD repair [14].

However, the early years of extracorporeal support were rife with error. In Lillehei's review of cardiac surgery performed between 1951 and 1954, he found that six centers had attempted procedures on 18 different patients. Of these 18 patients, only 1 survived, though there were many word-of-mouth reports speculating that many more unreported attempts were made. Of these 18, there was much diversity in the types of oxygenators used, from bubble to monkey lung and film [15]. This lack of uniformity was reflective of the infancy of the technology that necessitated each center not only to create their own device but also to navigate their own inexperience with actually using extracorporeal support and learning how the patients would interface with these novel devices. Aspects widely taken for granted today, such as steps of cannulation and de-airing, were still being learned, and standardized cannulae and sutures were still being developed. In addition, these rudimentary direct-contact heart-lung machines caused a fair amount of blood trauma, and postoperative coagulopathy was ubiquitous owing to the contact of the blood with air, metal, plastic, etc. Besides this, the longer the duration of extracorporeal support, the higher the incidence of other complications such as capillary leak, shock, and acidosis with progressive multiorgan failure, all of which forced clinicians to find work-arounds to limit the patient's exposure to these machines.

Largely, these temporizing solutions were either expeditious procedures or temperature management. At the time, the vast majority of centers were employing deep hypothermia (>15 degrees centigrade), which allowed perfusion to be ceased for up to 1 h [16]. Others were employing a novel technique during cooling, which employed separate right and left heart bypasses using the native lungs for oxygenation [17]. Regardless, these limitations and adaptations made use of these extracorporeal techniques untenable for longer term support of patients in the way we have come to employ in the critically ill, which would be ushered in with the development of the membrane oxygenator.

In 1944, Kolff and Berk published a description of a hemodialysis machine that consisted of 20,000 cm2 in which there was gas exchange between the blood and the aerated dialysate via passive diffusion [18]. This report showed the possibility of transferring gas without the need for blood to be indirect contact with air, thus limiting the issues seen with other direct-contact oxygenators. However, first there were engineering limitations that would need to be overcome. Chiefly, the sourcing of reasonable materials that were mechanically strong while being thin and permeable enough for gas exchange was the initial limitation to further development of this technology. However, as the production of synthetic materials grew in volume and techniques for synthesizing these became more efficient, materials such as polyethylene available. Kolff and Baltzer used this polyethylene rolled into a coil for their first publication of their success creating a membrane oxygenator, in this case a coil [19], though the design would eventually evolve to involve Teflon as the base material. Clowes, Hopkins, and Neville continued this work and in 1956 published a review of various synthetic materials and configurations to describe their mechanical strength and ability to transfer gas via a membrane composed of sandwiched membranes through which blood flows [20].

Following these descriptors, this group employed their design in experimental models using dogs and subsequently humans with remarkable results. They found that not only were they able to sustain life for prolonged periods, but they were also able to do so with less evidence of blood trauma, less malperfusion, and generally less complications [21]. Now that the possibility of membrane oxygenation had been established, much of the work in the coming years would focus on refinement and optimization of the technology prior to settling on thin layers of silicone covering nylon screens and sandwiched together. The use of silicone further reduced blood trauma by eliminating plasma loss, though the permeability being much higher for oxygen than for CO2 necessitated higher gas flow rates [22]. This gas exchange was dependent on the difference of partial pressures on either side of the membrane; thus, higher flow rates would ensure lower partial pressures on the gas side of the membrane. However, the layer of blood immediately in contact with the membrane would much more quickly equilibrate with the gas medium than the layers of blood deeper to the membrane. Thus, it was shown that the limiting factor in gas exchange was now the thickness of the blood layer [23]. In our lungs, the alveolar capillaries are a single red blood cell thick, allowing for ultraefficient gas exchange across the alveolar membrane. However, in artificial membranes, these blood channels are much larger, which was the emphasis of much work in the early 1960s seeking to minimize the size of these channels and optimize gas exchange.

The culmination of this effort resulted in the movement away from a membrane in the traditional sense and towards a sort of capillary formation of hollow silicone tubes with miniscule diameters (100–500 um) [24]. This configuration meant a smaller distance between blood layers and the surface of the membrane where gas exchange occurs, as well as the ability to better regulate the volumes of blood and gas on either side of the membrane.

Current State of Evidence

VV

Now that the problem of time limitation and effective gas transfer had been solved, it was possible to envision a time where this extracorporeal support would be able to be utilized outside of the surgical arena and in the medical support of critically ill patients, namely, those patients with profound respiratory failure for whom mechanical ventilation was either detrimental or of little benefit. The proof of concept was first shown in 1965 when Rashkind and colleagues utilized a bubble oxygenator in an effort to support a moribund infant with respiratory failure [25]. Though this patient died, the group showed biochemical changes that indicated that with development, this was a feasible enterprise to pursue. Then in the 1970s, there were two pinnacle reports of the use of ECMO for patients with respiratory failure. The first in 1972 was in a 24-year-old man that suffered multisystem trauma resulting in an aortic injury that was repaired. Four days following this repair, he developed refractory respiratory failure (what we now term ARDS); despite mechanical ventilation, his condition continued to worsen, and thus, his care team cannulated him peripherally for use of the ECMO. This support lasted for 75 h during which his oxygenation improved, and he was successfully decannulated [26]. Following this breakthrough, Bartlett and his team published on their experience using venoarterial ECMO in the support of infants. In their series, there were 13 patients, with 4 of them surviving (postoperative cardiac failure, respiratory distress syndrome, meconium aspiration, and persistent fetal circulation) [27]. In these years, there were other centers beginning to experiment with clinical applications of ECMO support, though largely revolving around respiratory support. In 1976, Gille and Bagniewski published a retrospective analysis of ECMO usage over the prior 10 years [28]. Their dataset included 233 patients with respiratory failure cared for by 90 medical teams in 7 countries. Of the 76% of patients with potentially reversible insults, these authors reported a 15% rate of what they termed "favorable outcome." It should be noted, however, that a "favorable outcome" was a patient breathing room air 30 days after decannulation. These early successes, carried out by a small group of dedicated physicians, ushered in a new era of ECMO support and investigations.

The first major investigation into the efficacy of ECMO as a support mechanism was undertaken from 1975 to 1977. In this trial, 90 patients with acute respiratory failure across 9 centers were randomized to either conventional mechanical ventilation or the use of ECMO support. The results of this trial were underwhelming with four patients in each group surviving, correlating with a <10% survival [29]. While this was a groundbreaking effort in coordinating across multiple centers to study a relatively novel technique, there have been criticisms raised that may explain the underwhelming results; it did provide some valuable information. In regard to criticism, there is room to question the mechanical ventilation techniques used and whether they were standardized across patients. This is especially true in light of current ARDS literature. Additionally, the selection criteria may have excluded the highest and lowest risk individuals, introducing a selection bias. Third, this is a new technology, and the centers had varying degrees of experience with the technical aspects leading to a not insignificant number of deaths related to what we would now term "technical complications." Lastly, given the influenza pandemic of the time, a disproportionate number of participants likely were suffering a specific viral illness, which would not be reflective of other years [30]. Despite these limitations, there were some interesting lessons from the study. From defining the mortality of ARDS to the acknowledgement that inexperienced centers may not increase survival using a modality that was novel, there were valuable lessons taken from this initial study [31].

On the heels of this negative study came another disappointing investigation, this time of extracorporeal carbon dioxide removal (ECCO2R). ECCO2R relies on the native lungs to provide the required oxygenation while utilizing the ECMO membrane with high gas flows to eliminate CO2. In doing so, it is possible to employ ultralow tidal volume ventilation and a low minute ventilation in an effort to reduce barotrauma while focusing on alveolar recruitment. This also allowed for lower blood flow rates in the ECMO circuit as well as smaller membranes, which reduced the amount of blood trauma seen as well. This technique garnered attention through animal models and anecdotal clinical usage that purported reasonable benefit [32]. There were a handful of case series presented; one in 1986 enrolled 43 patients who had "severe respiratory failure of a parenchymal origin" and were being mechanically ventilated. These patients were cannulated for venovenous ECMO using low flows and high gas rates, with the mechanical ventilator set to minimize peak pressures (35–45 mmHg) and low frequencies (3–5 breaths per minute). Remarkably, these authors showed improvement in lung function in 73% of the patients with 48% surviving, concluding that ECCO2R was a safe technique that may be an alternative technique to conventional mechanical ventilation [33]. However, disappointment came with the results of another randomized trial in 1994 with 40 patients enrolled to either conventional means of ARDS therapy or lung-protective inverse ratio ventilation with ECCO2R support. These authors found no difference in 30-day survival or oxygenation, leading them to conclude that ECCO2R could not be recommended as an alternative or adjunctive therapy [34].

These two negative trials had a chilling effect on investigations in ECMO use for adults. However, in a dichotomous fashion, work in pediatrics and specifically neonates was flourishing with positive results. As with adults, these investigations began as case series or anecdotal reports followed by studies with somewhat flawed designs and ultimately reasonably high-quality randomized trials. Dorson and his colleagues appreciated the special challenges inherent in providing extracorporeal support to infants. He postulated that such a device would need to require low priming volume, have little blood trauma, minimize exposed surface area, and have a short blood transit time [35]. Then, 2 years later in 1971, there came the first reports of infants being supported for a prolonged period, albeit without much long-term success [36]. Shortly after this, Bartlett and his group published their successful experience supporting an infant with meconium aspiration after which they published follow-up reports summarizing their experience. The first, in 1977, was composed of 12 neonates with respiratory distress from a myriad of pathology. This, largely a proof of concept, showed that ECMO could be beneficial though it did have some common complications, namely intracranial bleeding—albeit at lower rates with higher survival than with conventional ventilation [37]. In the following 5 years, Bartlett and his group treated 45 neonates for a heterogeneous group of pathologies (meconium aspiration, hyaline membrane disease, sepsis, and persistent fetal circulation) with good success. They reported a 50% survival rate which compelled centers to take notice and form their own ECMO teams [38].

These early successes compelled groups to continue pursuing these therapies and resulted in many neonatal centers then developing their own ECMO teams. These 18 centers then published their experience with over 700 patients, which showed a great success for ECMO being used to support neonates. This case series presented data over the previous 7 years, which showed an astounding 81% survival rate for all patients. The bulk of this benefit was seen in cases of meconium aspiration, where there was a reported 91% survival of the over 300 patients who were supported with ECMO. The lowest survival group was those with congenital diaphragmatic hernia, though even this group showed a 65% survival rate. Beyond adding support for the use of ECMO, this case series showed one other interesting point. Experience mattered—in this series, the average survival for the first 10 vs. the next 10 patients at any given center was 73% vs. 83% showing that there was a learning curve in establishing a system of care for these patients. Somewhat interestingly, this survival did not change for the following 20 patients however. Ultimately, the authors concluded that lung rest and support with ECMO were an "appropriate and successful treatment for newborn respiratory failure unresponsive to other forms of management" [39].

In the context of these case series showing compelling successes, work began on the first randomized controlled trials in pediatric ECMO use. The first trial enrolled 12 patients >2 kg and with high predicted mortality related to their respiratory failure, in an interesting "play the winner" randomization scheme. This meant that each subsequent patient was randomized based on how the others had performed before them. Thus, treatments with high rates of success would have more patients randomized to them. This drew post-publication criticism, however, as this resulted in a control group of 1 patient being randomized to conventional therapies and 11 randomized to receive ECMO support and lung rest at a time when ECMO was largely considered experimental. Despite this, there was a compelling statement made when all 11 ECMO patients survived (though 1 suffered intracerebral hemorrhage) and the lone conventional treatment patient died [40]. Growing on this work, a group from Boston sought to enroll more patients while avoiding some of the methodological criticisms. This trial enrolled 39 patients with persistent pulmonary hypertension and respiratory failure of the newborn, with the randomization ceased after the death of the fourth conventional medical therapy patient; in the end, 29 infants were randomized to ECMO support, with 28 of them surviving compared to 4 out of 10 infants in the conventional therapy arm dying [41].

While these single-center studies were interesting and drove the advancement and utility of ECMO, they were still single center and relatively small. This changed in 1996 when a group from the UK published the first multicenter randomized clinical trial of ECMO in neonatal respiratory failure involving 195 patients with enrollment stopped early due to a clear benefit being shown in the ECMO group. In this group, only 30 of the 92 patients died compared to 54 of the 92 conventional management group, with this benefit extending to the first year and showing less disability as well [42]. Additionally, there was a follow-up of these patients done 4 years after their initial enrollment, which did show slightly higher morbidity in the ECMO group largely related to neurocognitive complications from carotid cannulation though preserving the superiority of ECMO in terms of "death or severe disability" leading the authors to conclude that there was benefit to implementing ECMO as a policy in the treatment and support of patients with neonatal respiratory failure and that this essentially equated to one child saved for every four to five referred for ECMO [43].

Around this time, there continued to be growing interest in extrapolating the neonatal experience into the care of adults with respiratory failure. And, despite a negative trial in 1979, these positive studies in the pediatric arena continued to bolster support for the use of ECMO in adults. Following the negative results from Morris, much of the large-scale work had ceased though centers in Europe and the USA continued to publish their limited experiences. In 1997, a group in Germany published compelling data showing improved survival using an algorithm for treating ARDS that included entry points for patients to receive VV ECMO. In this study, they enrolled 122 sequential patients meeting ARDS criteria. Seventy-three of these patients received advanced noninvasive therapies, while 49 met either fast or slow criteria for receiving VV ECMO support resulting in an overall survival rate of 75% (89% survival in the non-ECMO group and 55% in the ECMO group). These results suggested not only that a patient care algorithm including ECMO may result in higher than expected survival, but also that the use of ECMO in select patients improves survival given the expected mortality in the ECMO group being upwards of 90% based on previous work [44]. That same year, a group from the USA published their recent experience supporting 141 patients with acute respiratory failure. In a similar fashion to the group from Germany, this group had one population that did not require VV ECMO initiation; in this case, 41 patients were referred to their center but made improvements so that they no longer qualified, as well as a group that met the criteria for initiation. The overall survival was 62% with 62 of the 100 ECMO patients being able to be weaned and 54 of them surviving to discharge [45]. In essence, this US group corroborated the experience from Germany with similar survival rates and showing a similar impact of ECMO on survival in specific populations.

Case series and publications such as these continued through the 1990s and early 2000s and evolved into a multicenter randomized controlled trial from the UK in 2009. Commonly known as the CESAR trial, this trial enrolled 180 adult patients with respiratory failure meeting the criteria (Murray score > 3 or hypercapnia with pH < 7.2) and randomized them to either continued conventional management or referral to an ECMO center for consideration of ECMO support. Overall, this resulted in 63% of those referred surviving without significant disability at 6 months compared to 47% that were not [46]. Critics of this study point out that only 2/3 of those referred for ECMO consideration ever received ECMO support, which does suggest that the benefit seen was not exclusively in the utility of ECMO but similar to prior case series being treated at a center where ECMO is part of the algorithm. Additionally, this study looked at cost, which not surprisingly showed an increased cost and length of stay [47]. However, the disability-free survival shown was compelling enough to drive the development of ECMO centers around the world. The result of CESAR, that patients with severe respiratory failure had increased survival at centers capable of offering ECMO, was seen again following the 2009 H1N1 pandemic, which provided an opportunity to increase experience and knowledge of how ECMO may benefit adults.

In an observational study from Australia and New Zealand, authors published their experience treating 201 patients with influenza that had developed severe ARDS. These 201 patients were treated at ECMO centers where 68 patients were supported with VV ECMO and 133 received conventional ARDS therapy, and the overall survival rate from 79% with a VV ECMO survival rate of 77% and a non-ECMO survival rate of 87% [48]. It is important to note that the patients receiving ECMO were not randomized, but instead initiation was based on clinical factors; thus, this group was sicker than the conventional therapy group. Their group had worse lung compliance reflected in higher airway pressures, higher PEEP, and worse gas exchange with higher PaCO2 and lower PaO2. As with prior work, this group had longer ICU stays and longer duration of mechanical ventilation. This experience was able to replicate findings from CESAR that patients treated at ECMO centers would have better outcomes while showing that for patients failing conventional therapy, ECMO was a valid option that may increase odds of survival. Groups in France and the UK published similar works with the French experience showing similar survival between those treated with ECMO and conventional therapies, albeit again with sicker patients receiving ECMO support [49]. The UK group had similar findings as CESAR and the French group that referral to an ECMO-capable center resulted in higher survival rates and that salvage ECMO may increase survival in this patient population albeit at the cost of increased length of stay [50]. These studies made a compelling statement that ARDS management in an algorithmic fashion that includes entry points for VV ECMO support increases survival and that the use of VV ECMO as a salvage for those patients failing traditional therapies likely increases the survival of these patients.

Expanding on CESAR was the EOLIA trial in 2018, which not only looked to substantiate the beneficial effects of having an algorithm with VV ECMO as an option, but also sought to introduce the question of timing of ECMO into the conversation. Up until this point, ECMO had largely been viewed as a rescue maneuver reserved for those patients in extremis that were failing traditional therapies. In this way, there was a suspicion that patients were being intervened upon at a time point too far into the disease course and only after complications from mechanical ventilation had begun to manifest. To this end, the authors of EOLIA randomized 249 patients across 64 European centers, all of which met the criteria for severe ARDS to either early application of ECMO or continued medical therapy with the ability to cross over to the ECMO group at a later point. There were 35 patients that did cross over, after having $SpO2 < 80\%$ for 6 h despite protocolized medical therapies. The trial was stopped early (75% enrollment) due to perceived futility as the authors were not showing a significant benefit of the ECMO arm. However, this is with some major criticisms. First, the study was vastly underpowered given the benefit the authors were trying to show and the mortality actually achieved in the control group (48%) being lower than hypothesized. Second, the crossing over of 35 patients (20 of which died and 9 of which were emergent VA cannulation during CPR) potentially diluted the effect of ECMO. And, third, this trial recruited patients over a 6-year period, which may capture practice changes. Overall, this trial provides evidence of the safety of ECMO use that at a minimum, it did not increase the mortality of patients unresponsive to traditional therapies and at its best shows some benefit of earlier initiation of ECMO in patients with profound hypoxic respiratory failure [51].

In 2020, the world found itself engulfed in a pandemic like it had never seen before. COVID-19, another respiratory viral illness, was ravaging communities and resulting in profound respiratory failure. Early in the pandemic, centers were publishing their experience with VV ECMO in supporting patients with refractory respiratory failure as the result of COVID-19 infection. Data from France, compiled at a single center using a matched cohort design enrolling almost 500 patients, 80 of which received VV ECMO support, showed survival figures that were at a minimum consistent with recent work in the non-COVID ARDS patient suggesting that ECMO remained a valuable tool in the treatment of refractory ARDS patient [52]. Later in 2020, The Lancet published an evaluation of the Extracorporeal Life Support Organization (ELSO) dataset from January through May of that year in which 1035 patients were supported with VV ECMO. These patients were cared for in 213 centers across 36 countries and represented the earliest patients with COVID to receive extracorporeal support. This cohort was relatively ill with a median P:F ratio of 72 mmHg and 60–70% of them receiving prone positioning and/or neuromuscular blockade prior to initiation of VV ECMO. Remarkably, the patients receiving ECMO support showed a 63% survival rate, further supporting the use of ECMO as support for those with respiratory failure refractory to conventional therapies [53]. This survival rate was further corroborated in 2022 in a meta-analysis with 4044 patients receiving ECMO support for COVID-19-related ARDS. These authors showed that while mortality was higher than compared to ECMO used in support of patients suffering influenza, it was sufficiently low to warrant further use [54].

One factor affecting the outcome of these patients who were on ECMO support during the COVID-19 pandemic appeared to be that of experience. Barbaro et al. also found that early-adopting centers showed lower 90-day mortality than late-adopting centers, and this was related to volume [55]. This also suggests that there is an opportunity to pool resources between centers and to transfer patients to higher volume centers when able.

ECMO for Cardiac Failure

Clearly, there is a benefit to managing patients with hypoxic respiratory failure using an algorithm that contains an entry point for VV ECMO support. Now, what of those patients with cardiac failure requiring temporary mechanical support? These patients, while a heterogeneous population of etiologies, generally fall into one of the three categories: heart failure, ECMO during CPR (ECPR), or temporary support due to obstructive shock (pulmonary embolism). Classically, venoarterial ECMO (VA-ECMO) has been used for postcardiotomy cardiogenic shock or those unable to wean from cardiopulmonary bypass in the operating room and may be performed via either central or peripheral cannulation. One recent multicenter retrospective cohort analysis of postcardiotomy cardiogenic shock showed relatively high mortality rates of 64.4% in hospital and 67.2% at 1 year, suggesting that these patients generally died in the hospital and if surviving to discharge did very well [56]. These authors additionally added to the conversation regarding experience by showing that those centers performing over 50 patients with postcardiotomy VA-ECMO showed significantly improved survival rates (60.9% vs. 70.2%) compared to centers treating fewer patients during the study period.

More recently, attention has been paid to the role that VA-ECMO plays in the resuscitation of patients suffering cardiac arrest. Out-of-hospital cardiac arrest is a condition with relatively high prevalence in North America and Europe, with an incidence of roughly 50 per 100,000, and is largely related to a cardiac etiology [57]. Despite many advances in medical therapies, the survival rates for cardiac arrest remain low at 10.7% globally, with the bulk of these survivors coming from those with cardiac arrest while in hospital as opposed to out of hospital [58]. As an effort to sustain life and support the patient until investigations can reveal reversible causes, VA-ECMO has been employed in an emergent fashion and with promising results. A group from Paris published their experience with ECPR use in OHCA, and it was the first large-scale experience to be shared. Their work showed a clear benefit of higher rates of favorable neurologic outcomes in patients receiving ECPR prior to hospital arrival compared to those being placed on ECMO after arrival, though there was no overall reduction in mortality in the ECMO cohort [59]. This lack of overall benefit may question the utility of ECPR though it is important to note that this study did not protocolize the use of VA-ECMO and instead left it to clinician discretion, and the patient population included both shockable and non-shockable rhythms. This has been studied further, and it was found that survival does differ between those with and those without shockable rhythms at the time of ECPR initiation compared with those with shockable rhythms having higher rates of survival [60]. In fact, one group from America has developed a mobile ECMO team that responds to patients in cardiac arrest with shockable rhythms. Over the course of 4 months in 2020, this team treated 63 patients, with 58 of them meeting the criteria and being placed on VA-ECMO during their resuscitation. These authors showed favorable functional outcome in 43% of patients enrolled, suggesting ECPR as a valuable tool in the management of refractory cardiac arrest [61]. The role of ECMO in cardiac arrest continues to be investigated with promising results.

Current State of the ECMO Community

These continued developments and investigations with promising results continue to move the field forward. As experience continues to grow and interest in ECMO for respiratory and/or cardiac failure gains traction, there has been a growth in centers and organizations around the world. Leading the way in this growth is the pre-eminent professional society for the use of extracorporeal life support, Extracorporeal Life Support Organization (ELSO). ELSO was formed in 1989 as a voluntary alliance of the main centers at that time. Prior to this, in the mid-1980s, there were only three centers regularly utilizing ECMO for life support—University of Michigan, University of Pittsburgh, and Medical College of Virginia. Smaller programs were being developed, though at the time there was no social media or Internet to drive development, and these new centers largely came about through movement of experienced faculty to new institutions and relied heavily on the mentorship of these more experienced institutions. By the late 1980s, at the time of the alliance being formed, upwards of 20 centers in the USA were performing ECMO. Eventually, this alliance led to the first international meeting of this newly formed professional society, which drew international interest. This subsequently led to the development of the European group of ELSO, European Extracorporeal Life Support Organization (EESO).

These organizations have worked together to not only compile robust datasets around the growing volume of ECMO yearly, but also collaborate and develop best practices and guidelines for centers to reference for their own programs and management. Out of this grew the "Red Book" which is the collaboration of experts from various centers aiming to provide concise and evidence-based recommendations for ECMO management and program development. The database that was created continues to grow each year with upwards of 100,000 patient cases and not only allows centers to compare their outcomes to the greater ECMO community but also provides a dataset for investigating outcomes as they relate to indication or other variables.

In 2021, there were over 170,000 ECMO cases worldwide, representing continued growth and an embrace of extracorporeal modalities in the support of the critically ill. In the 92 years since Dr. Gibbon lay awake at night, fretting over the powerless feeling of watching a young woman die from pulmonary embolism, there has been amazing advancements in this field of extracorporeal support. Starting with the discovery that blood could be oxygenated without the use of the lungs and culminating in the modern hollow fiber oxygenators, physicians and scientists were able to solve the problem of gas exchange not relying on the patient's lungs. In parallel, engineers worked to develop a machine that would be able to remove and reinfuse blood from patients with minimal blood trauma, now represented by the modern magnetically levitated and frictionless pump heads in common use. Around the USA and subsequently the globe, physicians and centers have banded together to share their mutually beneficial experiences, successes, and failures, to collaborate at improving the outcomes of patients.

References

1. Bartlett RH, John H, Lecture GJ. Extracorporeal life support: Gibbon fulfilled. J Am Coll Surg. 2014;218:317–27.
2. Clark LC Jr, Gollan F, Gupta VB. The oxygenation of blood by gas dispersion. Science. 1950;111:85–7.
3. Björk VO. Brain perfusions in dogs with artificially oxygened blood. Lund: Berlingska Boktryck; 1948.
4. Gibbon JH Jr. Application of a mechanical heart and lung apparatus to cardiac surgery. Minn Med. 1954;37:171–85; passim.
5. Dr. mustard's macabre monkey machine by Gary grist and Kelly Hedlund. In: Perfusion theory [Internet]. 30 Dec 2021 [cited 20 Dec 2022]. Available: https://perfusiontheory.com/history/dr-mustards-macabre-monkey-machine-by-gary-grist-and-kelly-hedlund/
6. Cross FS, Berne RM, Hirose Y, Jones RD, Kay EB. Evaluation of a rotating disc type reservoir-oxygenator. Proc Soc Exp Biol Med. 1956;93:210–4.
7. McLean J. The discovery of heparin. Circulation. 1959;19:75–8.
8. Ransdell HT Jr, Haller JA Jr, Stowens D, Barton PB. Renal toxicity of polybrene, (hexadimethrine bromide). J Surg Res. 1965;5:195–9.
9. Hewitt RL, Creech O Jr. History of the pump oxygenator. Arch Surg. 1966;93:680–96.
10. Lillehei CW, Dewall RA, Read RC, Warden HE, Varco RL. Direct vision intracardiac surgery in man using a simple, disposable artificial oxygenator. Dis Chest. 1956;29:1–8.
11. Lillehei CW, Varco RL, Cohen M, Warden HE, Patton C, Moller JH. The first open-heart repairs of ventricular septal defect, atrioventricular communis, and tetralogy of Fallot using extracorporeal circulation by cross-circulation: a 30-year follow-up. Ann Thorac Surg. 1986;41:4–21.
12. Iles TL, Holm MA, Calvin AD, Moller JH, Iaizzo PA. First successful open-heart surgery utilizing cross-circulation in 1954. Ann Thorac Surg. 2020;110:336–41.
13. Wert R. How a car company built the world's first mechanical heart. In: Jalopnik [Internet]. 20 Jul 2011 [cited 22 Dec 2022]. Available: https://jalopnik.com/how-a-car-company-built-the-worlds-first-mechanical-hea-5822972

14. Hill JD, John H, Gibbon J, Part I. The development of the first successful heart-lung machine. Ann Thorac Surg. 1982;34:337–41.
15. Gravlee GP. Cardiopulmonary bypass: principles and practice. Philadelphia: Lippincott Williams & Wilkins; 2008.
16. Hurt R. The technique and scope of open-heart surgery. Postgrad Med J. 1967;43:668–74.
17. Drew CE, Anderson IM. Profound hypothermia in cardiac surgery: report of three cases. Lancet. 1959;1:748–50.
18. Kolff WJ, Berk HTJ, Welle NM. The artificial kidney: a dialyser with a great area. Scandinavica. 1944. Available: https://onlinelibrary.wiley.com/doi/abs/10.1111/j.0954-6820.1944.tb03951.x?casa_token=EsC3Y5ydnm4AAAAA:Pgkx6-6GaQ86Kj1dV YLw-UGty_KLF1VVNOu0Kw3KhxU0fZBcqm6HGN61cdc37BaF5S2ZbWt9brJBWGw
19. Kolff WJ, Balzer R, Cleveland MD. The artificial coil lung. ASAIO J. 1955;1:39.
20. Clowes GH Jr, Hopkins AL, Neville WE. An artificial lung dependent upon diffusion of oxygen and carbon dioxide through plastic membranes. J Thorac Surg. 1956;32:630–7.
21. Clowes GHA Jr, Neville WE. Further development of a blood oxygenator dependent upon the diffusion of gases through plastic membranes. ASAIO J. 1957;3:52.
22. Kammermeyer K. Silicone rubber as a selective barrier. Ind Eng Chem. 1957;49:1685–6.
23. Marx TI, Snyder WE, St John AD, Moeller CE. Diffusion of oxygen into a film of whole blood. J Appl Physiol. 1960;15:1123–9.
24. Bodell BR, Head JM, Head LR, Formolo AJ, Head JR. A capillary membrane oxygenator. J Thorac Cardiovasc Surg. 1963;46:639–50.
25. Rashkind WJ, Freeman A, Klein D, Toft RW. Evaluation of a disposable plastic, low volume, pumpless oxygenator as a lung substitute. J Pediatr. 1965;66:94–102.
26. Hill JD, O'Brien TG, Murray JJ, Dontigny L, Bramson ML, Osborn JJ, et al. Prolonged extracorporeal oxygenation for acute post-traumatic respiratory failure (shock-lung syndrome). Use of the Bramson membrane lung. N Engl J Med. 1972;286:629–34.
27. Bartlett RH, Gazzaniga AB, Jefferies MR, Huxtable RF, Haiduc NJ, Fong SW. Extracorporeal membrane oxygenation (ECMO) cardiopulmonary support in infancy. Trans Am Soc Artif Intern Organs. 1976;22:80–93.
28. Gille JP, Bagniewski AM. Ten years of use of extracorporeal membrane oxygenation (ECMO) in the treatment of acute respiratory insufficiency (ARI). Trans Am Soc Artif Intern Organs. 1976;22:102–9.
29. Zapol WM, Snider MT, Hill JD, Fallat RJ, Bartlett RH, Edmunds LH, et al. Extracorporeal membrane oxygenation in severe acute respiratory failure. A randomized prospective study. JAMA. 1979;242:2193–6.
30. Lim MW. The history of extracorporeal oxygenators. Anaesthesia. 2006;61:984–95.
31. Bartlett RH. Extracorporeal life support: history and new directions. Semin Perinatol. 2005;29:2–7.
32. Kolobow T, Gattinoni L, Tomlinson T, Pierce JE. An alternative to breathing. J Thorac Cardiovasc Surg. 1978;75:261–6.
33. Gattinoni L, Pesenti A, Mascheroni D, Marcolin R, Fumagalli R, Rossi F, et al. Low-frequency positive-pressure ventilation with extracorporeal CO2 removal in severe acute respiratory failure. JAMA. 1986;256:881–6.
34. Morris AH, Wallace CJ, Menlove RL, Clemmer TP, Orme JF Jr, Weaver LK, et al. Randomized clinical trial of pressure-controlled inverse ratio ventilation and extracorporeal CO2 removal for adult respiratory distress syndrome. Am J Respir Crit Care Med. 1994;149:295–305.
35. Dorson W Jr, Baker E, Cohen ML, Meyer B, Molthan M, Trump D, et al. A perfusion system for infants. Trans Am Soc Artif Intern Organs. 1969;15:155–60.
36. White JJ, Andrews HG, Risemberg H, Mazur D, Haller JA Jr. Prolonged respiratory support in newborn infants with a membrane oxygenator. Surgery. 1971;70:288–96.
37. Bartlett RH, Gazzaniga AB, Huxtable RF, Schippers HC, O'Connor MJ, Jefferies MR. Extracorporeal circulation (ECMO) in neonatal respiratory failure. J Thorac Cardiovasc Surg. 1977;74:826–33.

38. Bartlett RH, Andrews AF, Toomasian JM, Haiduc NJ, Gazzaniga AB. Extracorporeal membrane oxygenation for newborn respiratory failure: forty-five cases. Surgery. 1982;92:425–33.
39. Toomasian JM, Snedecor SM, Cornell RG, Cilley RE, Bartlett RH. National experience with extracorporeal membrane oxygenation for newborn respiratory failure. Data from 715 cases. ASAIO Trans. 1988;34:140–7.
40. Bartlett RH, Roloff DW, Cornell RG, Andrews AF, Dillon PW, Zwischenberger JB. Extracorporeal circulation in neonatal respiratory failure: a prospective randomized study. Pediatrics. 1985;76:479–87.
41. O'Rourke PP, Crone RK, Vacanti JP, Ware JH, Lillehei CW, Parad RB, et al. Extracorporeal membrane oxygenation and conventional medical therapy in neonates with persistent pulmonary hypertension of the newborn: a prospective randomized study. Pediatrics. 1989;84:957–63.
42. UK collaborative randomised trial of neonatal extracorporeal membrane oxygenation. UK Collaborative ECMO Trail Group. Lancet. 1996;348:75–82.
43. Bennett CC, Johnson A, Field DJ, Elbourne D, UK Collaborative ECMO Trial Group. UK collaborative randomised trial of neonatal extracorporeal membrane oxygenation: follow-up to age 4 years. Lancet. 2001;357:1094–6.
44. Lewandowski K, Rossaint R, Pappert D, Gerlach H, Slama KJ, Weidemann H, et al. High survival rate in 122 ARDS patients managed according to a clinical algorithm including extracorporeal membrane oxygenation. Intensive Care Med. 1997;23:819–35.
45. Kolla S, Awad SS, Rich PB, Schreiner RJ, Hirschl RB, Bartlett RH. Extracorporeal life support for 100 adult patients with severe respiratory failure. Ann Surg. 1997;226:544–64; discussion 565–6.
46. Peek GJ, Mugford M, Tiruvoipati R, Wilson A, Allen E, Thalanany MM, et al. Efficacy and economic assessment of conventional ventilatory support versus extracorporeal membrane oxygenation for severe adult respiratory failure (CESAR): a multicentre randomised controlled trial. Lancet. 2009;374:1351–63.
47. Zwischenberger JB, Lynch JE. Will CESAR answer the adult ECMO debate? Lancet. 2009;374:1307–8.
48. Australia and New Zealand Extracorporeal Membrane Oxygenation (ANZ ECMO) Influenza Investigators, Davies A, Jones D, Bailey M, Beca J, Bellomo R, et al. Extracorporeal membrane oxygenation for 2009 influenza A(H1N1) acute respiratory distress syndrome. JAMA. 2009;302:1888–95.
49. Roch A, Lepaul-Ercole R, Grisoli D, Bessereau J, Brissy O, Castanier M, et al. Extracorporeal membrane oxygenation for severe influenza A (H1N1) acute respiratory distress syndrome: a prospective observational comparative study. Intensive Care Med. 2010;36:1899–905.
50. Noah MA, Peek GJ, Finney SJ, Griffiths MJ, Harrison DA, Grieve R, et al. Referral to an extracorporeal membrane oxygenation center and mortality among patients with severe 2009 influenza A(H1N1). JAMA. 2011;306:1659–68.
51. Desai M, Dalton HJ. Half-empty or half-full?-interpretation of the EOLIA trial and thoughts for the future. J Thorac Dis. 2018;10:S3248–51.
52. Schmidt M, Hajage D, Lebreton G, Monsel A, Voiriot G, Levy D, et al. Extracorporeal membrane oxygenation for severe acute respiratory distress syndrome associated with COVID-19: a retrospective cohort study. Lancet Respir Med. 2020;8:1121–31.
53. Barbaro RP, MacLaren G, Boonstra PS, Iwashyna TJ, Slutsky AS, Fan E, et al. Extracorporeal membrane oxygenation support in COVID-19: an international cohort study of the extracorporeal life support organization registry. Lancet. 2020;396:1071–8.
54. Bertini P, Guarracino F, Falcone M, Nardelli P, Landoni G, Nocci M, et al. ECMO in COVID-19 patients: a systematic review and meta-analysis. J Cardiothorac Vasc Anesth. 2022;36:2700–6.
55. Barbaro RP, MacLaren G, Boonstra PS, Combes A, Agerstrand C, Annich G, et al. Extracorporeal membrane oxygenation for COVID-19: evolving outcomes from the international extracorporeal life support organization registry. Lancet. 2021;398:1230–8.

56. Biancari F, Dalén M, Fiore A, Ruggieri VG, Saeed D, Jónsson K, et al. Multicenter study on postcardiotomy venoarterial extracorporeal membrane oxygenation. J Thorac Cardiovasc Surg. 2020;159:1844–1854.e6.
57. Wong CX, Brown A, Lau DH, Chugh SS, Albert CM, Kalman JM, et al. Epidemiology of sudden cardiac death: global and regional perspectives. Heart Lung Circ. 2019;28:6–14.
58. Yan S, Gan Y, Jiang N, Wang R, Chen Y, Luo Z, et al. The global survival rate among adult out-of-hospital cardiac arrest patients who received cardiopulmonary resuscitation: a systematic review and meta-analysis. Crit Care. 2020;24:61.
59. Bougouin W, Dumas F, Lamhaut L, Marijon E, Carli P, Combes A, et al. Extracorporeal cardiopulmonary resuscitation in out-of-hospital cardiac arrest: a registry study. Eur Heart J. 2020;41:1961–71.
60. Fukushima K, Aoki M, Nakajima J, Aramaki Y, Ichikawa Y, Isshiki Y, et al. Favorable prognosis by extracorporeal cardiopulmonary resuscitation for subsequent shockable rhythm patients. Am J Emerg Med. 2022;53:144–9.
61. Bartos JA, Frascone RJ, Conterato M, Wesley K, Lick C, Sipprell K, et al. The Minnesota mobile extracorporeal cardiopulmonary resuscitation consortium for treatment of out-of-hospital refractory ventricular fibrillation: program description, performance, and outcomes. E Clin Med. 2020;29–30:100632.

Chapter 2
Program Development

Mark Caridi-Scheible ⓘ

Creating an ECMO Program

A distinction should be made between developing the capability to initiate and manage a patient on ECMO and a structured ECMO program. The first requires a minimum level of technical and medical knowledge and some baseline equipment. The remainder of this book is generally concerned with providing this competency. The second however includes all the activities and resources that allow the first to be successful and sustainable. Managing personnel, maintaining equipment, providing training, maintaining quality control and outcomes, controlling costs, managing referral networks, and marketing: these are just a few components of a structured program that can mean the difference between healthy growth of a program and its termination by hospital administration. While this chapter is mostly aimed at program leaders responsible for creating and maintaining the infrastructure of a program, it is also useful for any team member wanting to understand their own role in a program, how it relates to the greater effort of the team, and why certain decisions get made.

It should be said here that this chapter is largely based on expert opinion and cumulative experiences. There is a paucity of data as these are difficult studies to do rigorously. We will present some generalities to consider here, but in the absence of true data, there are also two further recommendations:

1. Unless you have prior experience, you should seek help and mentorship when starting a new program.

M. Caridi-Scheible (✉)
Division of Critical Care Medicine, Emory University School of Medicine, Atlanta, GA, USA
e-mail: mark.caridi-scheible@emory.edu

© The Author(s), under exclusive license to Springer Nature
Switzerland AG 2024
A. R. Taha et al. (eds.), *ECMO: A Practical Guide to Management*,
https://doi.org/10.1007/978-3-031-59634-6_2

2. Recognize that the Extracorporeal Life Support Organization (ELSO) maintains very detailed guidelines on the required components of an ECMO program both in their published guidelines [1] and in their specifications for ECMO Center of Excellence designation. In many localities, these guidelines may represent standard of care, and every practitioner should be familiar with them.

While there are no studies that directly demonstrate the superiority of a structured ECMO program, broad inferences can perhaps be made from such studies as PROSEVA [2] and CESAR [3] demonstrating that outcomes for a modality or diagnosis can be improved by centers of multidisciplinary care specifically skilled in that modality or diagnosis. It is conceivable for ECMO to run at an institution in an ad hoc fashion; however, this is difficult to grow and manage as there is no ownership or accountability [4]. Generally, ad hoc programs occur as an extension of a cardiothoracic surgery service line using equipment from the OR and other OR resources (e.g., perfusionists). This makes sense when the usage is restricted to a small subset of their own patients (say postcardiotomy or periprocedural patients). However, it can become unsustainable from surgeons' perspective when the indications become broader such as for respiratory failure, ECPR, advanced heart failure, and remote cannulation.

Table 2.1 summarizes the various types of ECMO program structures along with their advantages and disadvantages [5]. The structure for your particular program will depend on your institution's available resources, risk tolerance, local market demands, patient population, payer mix and reimbursement method, and staff interest. In general, however, the largest part of program development is in coordinating and developing internal expertise in physicians, affiliate providers (NPs and PAs), nurses, perfusionists, and respiratory therapists [6]. Developing good systems for training, outcome tracking, equipment management, and complication management also takes an enormous amount of time and effort and is best accomplished using a smaller number of patients to work out problems [7]. Paying a greater amount of attention to a smaller number of patients initially can also allow for better outcomes if the staff are relatively inexperienced, which is important when a young program is trying to improve itself. For all these reasons, it is almost always better for a program to start small and grow at an incremental rate. However, if the resources and experience are available, or else the market forces demand it, it is possible to jump directly to a larger program either with a large up-front investment or else by contracting out the services. A contractor would provide all the equipment and personnel required for the program and manage all the day-to-day operations in a turnkey manner.

Table 2.1 Summary of program types with pros and cons

Program type and number of patients	Pros	Cons
Ad hoc • OR or rented equipment and OR perfusionists • Primary provider provides all care	• Individual providers maintain tight control • Shared resources = low maintenance costs, particularly if low volume	• Lack of unified vision • Occupies resources meant for other settings (i.e., OR) • No systematic accountability for outcomes
Small start • 2–4 patients • Incremental growth (2–4/year) • Experienced program director • Experienced perfusionist • Program coordinator ideally, but may not need to be as experienced	• Lower entry costs • Lower initial burden on space and other fixed resources (nursing, etc.) • Can start with relatively inexperienced providers (physicians/PAs/NPs) and nurses • Allows for small-scale testing of in-house systems (education, QA, etc.) • Allows for more intense attention to a few patients as providers learn	• Slow growth may not meet market demands • Although lower initial capital expense, does lack economies of scale (for instance, volume discounts on disposables, labor flexing)
Large start • 8–10 patients • Incremental growth (resource dependent) • Very experienced program director • Experienced program coordinator • Experienced lead specialist or head perfusionists • Several experienced nurses	• Immediate economies of scale • Immediate ability to be market competitive and fulfill any referral network obligations	• High up-front costs in equipment, hiring, and training • Requires a core of experienced providers and nurses that can guide training of remainder of staff • Requires fully developed systems for education, management protocols, QA, budgeting, etc. Generally, these are brought in by hiring an experienced program director and coordinator
Contract out • Minimum patients set by contract agency • Resources depending on agency	• Highly flexible • Provides all protocols, education, etc. • Provides bedside management and support • Provides equipment • Can eventually transition to in-house management depending on terms of contract	• Expensive, but may be offset by lower short-term risk compared to large start option if this scale is required • Not available in all regions or countries

Program Structure and Management

There are a number of components to a successful program that we will discuss individually here, but they are all interrelated. Particularly in regard to staffing and equipment, there is a wide variety of configurations used in real practice, so it is important to pay attention here to the important minimum requirements.

Leadership

Program leadership is probably the greatest defining feature of an ECMO program as it introduces both directed management and accountability for success. At a minimum, a program director (PD) is required to set the goals for the programs and oversee their execution, delegating as able as the program grows and subleaders are added. The PD is a physician-level provider who can understand the underlying medical management, has a strong foundational knowledge of ECMO, and has working relationship with the various hospital administrators required to secure the resources that will be needed.

Since the PD likely has clinical and other duties and may not be able to manage the program daily at a low level, the recommended next step is the addition of an ECMO coordinator (EC) who really manages the program on a daily basis [8]. This is generally an affiliate-level provider (nurse practitioner, physician assistant) as it can be helpful for the person to have prescriptive authority, but depending on the institutional practice or requirements, this could also often be a nursing staff or even be a nonclinical person with sufficient experience. The EC's role can vary depending on the skill set and may be strictly administrative (data tracking, personnel management, educational program development, inventory management, and purchasing) to clinical (receiving consult calls, operative assist, daily rounding). As the responsibilities for the EC increase with program size, splitting the role into multiple positions may be required. This is a sufficiently critical role however that it is a requirement to obtain Center of Excellence designation from ELSO. In our experience, program growth was limited without a full-time person dedicated to managing the small day-to-day details of a larger program once moving beyond the 2–4 concurrent patient threshold.

Larger programs can yet further subdivide their programs into VA or VV components, perhaps separating surgical and medical directors, directors for education, eCPR, or cannulation. These will depend ultimately on how your groups function, who is cannulating, and who is managing which subset of patients and in which locations. The important point however is that they continue to be united by the program director into a cohesive program with a common set of goals, shared resources, and expectations for accountability.

The ECMO Team

ECMO is a team sport. It requires additional knowledge from and the coordinated efforts of everyone that touches the patient in order to be successful. Table 2.2 summarizes the various people that may be involved and their possible roles. Some are unique to the ECMO world and will be discussed in more detail. Sometimes, roles are fulfilled by the same person; for instance, a nurse may be both the bedside nurse and the specialist. These are institutional decisions, but the important thing is to

Table 2.2 Summary of roles and responsibilities within an ECMO program

Specialist	The bedside specialist is unique to the ECMO patient and is defined as the person responsible for the minute-to-minute management of the ECMO pump and circuit. This person must be immediately at hand in case of alarms and to handle emergencies such as pump failure. They also handle titrations within parameters set by the management team. They manage documentation and charting. Depending on the skill set of the person filling this position, they may cover a variable number of patients at a time, but must be in proximity to all of them. Management and training of the specialist team is potentially the most complicated personnel activity in the program and is discussed below.
Perfusionist	Perfusionists manage cardiopulmonary bypass machines in the OR for cardiac surgery, and it is a core part of their education and privileges to manage ECMO devices and circuits. The level of familiarity with specific devices may vary and their experience with long-term management in the ICU as well, but this is generally a matter of in-service training for them. As such, it is not uncommon for perfusionists to be used exclusively as specialists as the training overhead is low and they can often cover a greater number of patients with more confidence. However, they generally cost more and may have other duties in the OR. Regardless, at least one lead perfusionist is generally needed in a program to provide higher level consultation on equipment purchase decisions, complex configurations, equipment problems, and interface with the OR. They are also generally better suited for assisting with cannulation, particularly in a remote setting; however, this may depend on the skill of specialists and proceduralist comfort.
Critical care management	Patients on ECMO are by definition critically ill. Their outcomes depend on optimal medical management including nutrition, lung-protective ventilation, sepsis management, cardiac management, etc. A critical care medicine (CCM) team (physician and affiliate provider level) experienced in managing all the usual CCM issues, but in the setting of ECMO and the nuances involved, is important. The CCM team needs to be integrated and harmonized with the goals of the ECMO team. Increasingly, the CCM teams are specialized enough that they are handling the ECMO management as well, but it is still common that these are separate functions. The trend however is that bedside providers are expected to either have some fellowship training in ECMO management during their CCM fellowship or pursue some other training. Again, this is reflected in ELSO's Center of Excellence recommendations including continuing education for bedside providers. New programs should at the very least define the expectations for the level of training and plan for continuing education, even if it is minimal.

(continued)

Table 2.2 (continued)

ECMO management	This team consists of a physician provider and possible delegates (affiliate providers and trainees) who round daily on the patient and determine daily management goals for the ECMO circuit, anticoagulation goals, weaning, cannula maintenance, and revision. Often, particularly in VA-ECMO, this team is surgeon-led, and there are specific surgical goals intertwined with the ECMO care. These plans should be clearly communicated to the bedside specialist and to the CCM team (if different team). This team is generally often responsible for longitudinal care of the patient including follow-up on the floor or clinic for follow-up or stitch removal.
Cannulation	This team is a set of proceduralists who have trained specifically to place cannulas and initiate ECMO flows. Traditionally, this has been a cardiothoracic surgeon as it is already a core competency; however, as the technology and techniques have improved, it is increasingly common for intensivists, interventional cardiologists, interventional radiologists, and other proceduralists to be adept at vascular access to perform this role. There are arguments for and against various individuals performing the role, but no data argues for one over the other [9], and these are invariably institution dependent. What is invariable though is that all the individuals in a program performing cannulations should be performing it under a common set of guidelines using a common structure and shared understanding of the resources available. The most common pitfall is for those with access to the devices and ability to initiate, but not even remotely associated with the ECMO program, to give in to the temptation to cannulate a patient that by consensus of the ECMO team and its official policy would never have been a candidate. These are very difficult conversations to have with someone else's service, and it helps to have a prepared method of following up with your institution's administration. What can be helpful is to advocate for a formal institution-wide set of privileges the hospital requires in order to initiate ECMO.
Surgical support	Even if your cannulation and ECMO management team is entirely staffed with medicine-trained physicians, there is an inevitable and obligate amount of surgical support that ECMO patients will require. As the program numbers grow, complications will include vessel injuries, complex wound and intrathoracic problems, ischemic limbs, and VTE that will require a surgeon to correct. Tracheostomies are required. As programs grow in complexity (more VA-ECMO, transplant, nontraditional cannulation strategies), there is also necessary surgeon involvement. Understanding that this relationship is mutually beneficial and that a collaborative model is possible under most circumstances will make the process easier. But these relationships must be built early; particularly in smaller and more community institutions, there may be a great reluctance for more bread-and-butter surgeons (and the anesthesiologists) to get involved with what are often perceived as hopeless cases. The need to make friends, highlight positive outcomes, and emphasize a team approach cannot be overstated.

Table 2.2 (continued)

Nursing	With some exceptions, generally, the ECMO patients in the unit are the sickest of the sick. The nurses assigned to these patients need to be willing, dedicated, and experienced. It is strongly recommended that a 1:1 nurse-to-patient ratio be used. Additionally, there is some minimum amount of training with ECMO patients in general they should have. This need not be extensive, but is practical and needs to be maintained by a specified minimum amount of yearly contact with ECMO patients per year (as defined by your own institution). Some care points particular to the patient are cannula site care, turning the patient safely, basics of interpreting the hemodynamics, and titration goals that may be asked for. This is different from the bedside specialist, although in some institutions the nurse will be trained to serve both roles simultaneously (not recommended). However, nurses do make good bedside specialists as a distinct role from their nursing duties with appropriate training.
Respiratory therapy	Respiratory therapists (RTs) who manage vents or other respiratory devices in the ECMO setting have to have some familiarity with the different goals while on ECMO. If there is no inclusion of the RT team in the ECMO program, then there needs to be a very clear understanding and mechanism for communicating vent orders and other respiratory orders that are not modifiable without the ECMO team's awareness. Often, it is better to have the RT team be an integral part and receive training so they understand the physiology and rationale behind the demands. Even better is to train them as bedside specialists if that is the model your program uses.
Physical therapy	Early physical therapy (PT) and mobilization are known to improve outcomes in multiple postsurgical studies and ICU studies, and ECMO is no different. As will be described elsewhere in this book, patients on ECMO whenever possible should be awake and mobilized. Although cannulation strategy may impose some limits, PT should always be under consideration by a PT team experienced in working around those limitations. It will take time for the existing hospital's PT team to develop the skills required to work with ECMO patients, and there is even a growing set of PT literature dedicated to this. Engage this team early, and identify individuals who are willing and excited to become these experts.

understand the activities that these people perform and to ensure that it is clear every day and every hour that all the tasks are accounted for by a defined person. This is not a trivial statement. Particularly for smaller programs with more limited resources, personnel is often the limiting factor. However, a program must be able to guarantee without fail that a trained specialist will be at the bedside 24 h a day to manage the circuit and that if an emergency happens and that person cannot, there is an emergency plan (for instance, an on-call perfusionist, or the program director sits pump). If these backup plans are not viable, then the program should not be operating. That is only one example. A viable program needs to make sure that all of the following roles and tasks are adequately and sustainably covered (Table 2.2).

The Bedside Specialist

As described in Table 2.2, the bedside specialist is a unique and critical role that absolutely must be present in some form 24 h a day, 7 days a week, without fail. When that person must be absent for meals or breaks, a backup person must be present. The specific person occupying this role may have other concomitant roles (not recommended) or have different base skill sets (perfusionist, nurse, respiratory therapist, affiliate provider, physician). Regardless of base profession, all specialists need to have the same training and experience in managing a defined set of tasks and emergencies. This should be guaranteed by a structured training and orientation and then by a regular assessment of competency (usually yearly). The expected competencies for a specialist are well delineated by ELSO in their guidelines.

The choice of base profession to fill the role is driven by local availability and experience and by economic considerations for the particular institution. Therefore, although it is possible for a physician or affiliate-level provider to fill this role, and this may make sense for emergencies or startup phases of a program, it is generally not cost-effective. This generally leaves three different models that are used, summarized in Table 2.3. The first employs the nurse that is already in the room to also manage the circuit at the same time with no additional personnel to help. The second uses perfusionists alone as specialists. The third uses either nurses or respiratory therapists, or both, operating outside of their usual roles and performing only the tasks of managing the pump and circuit for one or more patients.

Table 2.3 Summary of bedside staffing models

Model	Pros	Cons
Room nurse only	• Cost-effective	• Requires experienced nurses • Nurse burnout • Nurses already overburdened with tasks for sick patients (e.g., CRRT)
Perfusionist only	• Generally more comfortable monitoring many more pumps simultaneously (1:6–10) • Cost-effective at higher patient ratios • Low training overhead • Highly skilled at baseline, better with more complex patients (e.g., VAV, VADs with oxygenators) • Can participate in procedures and advanced troubleshooting	• Lower supply • More expensive for lower patient ratios
Separate nurse or RT	• Cost-balanced when operating at the high end of ratios • Can be used as retention tool for career development and additional pay opportunity • Both have roughly same training overhead	• Diverts nursing and RT resources in times of shortages • In times of shortages, may have to run with higher ratios than desired or use backup perfusionists. Need to have a plan

The ratio of specialist to patients is dependent on the experience of the specialists and the complexity of the ECMO patients, but 1:3 is a common ratio meaning larger programs that exceed their set ratio will require additional specialists be concurrently available. The pros and cons of each of these models are summarized in Table 2.3. Because perfusionists come essentially already trained, it is often the case that a program will start with perfusionists at the bedside while they train a team of specialists and let them orient with the perfusionists. This can take many months to years to complete this transition but allows time to develop a robust and large pool of specialists without burning out the few at the beginning. Additionally, for larger programs, a hybrid model may also be indicated where perfusionists perhaps take care of more complex patients and nurse/RT specialists take care of lower ratio of more straightforward.

Consults

An ECMO program needs patients that require ECMO, and this requires having a defined set of criteria about what that patient looks like and then marketing those criteria both internally and externally so your colleagues can refer you qualified patients. This process takes effort. The first step is to establish your criteria which should be well defined and consistent. All of your colleagues that take consult calls with you should be in general agreement so that referrers do not view your institution as confusing or unpredictable (assuming they have a choice).

The next step is to make it known that the service is available and have a method to make it happen. Internally, this might be as simple as a presentation to the intensivist group or the cardiology group with contact numbers or pagers for calling a consult as you would any other consult. Externally, you should start by registering your site with ELSO as an ECMO center. Then make sure that your transfer center (or whatever operator service receives requests to transfer patients to you) is aware of your service line and has an on-call number to talk to an ECMO consultant. It may also be a good idea to call the unit directors for surrounding area hospitals to let them know that you are accepting transfers for possible ECMO patients.

It is perhaps surprising to many that competing ECMO centers are actually quite cooperative with each other. In times of stress, particularly during the pandemic, spare circuits were shared when there were shortages, patients were load-balanced when capacity was full, educational efforts are shared, and the list goes on. ECMO really is a small community, and there is plenty of volume to go around. It is a good idea as a new program to make contact with surrounding programs to enable these kind of cooperative efforts.

Lastly, as you build your referral network, never take it for granted. Even internally, repeat business relies on a positive perception of you by the customers (referring physicians). They want to see consistency, respect, concern for their patients, and a willingness to help even if ECMO is not the solution. It is worth investing the extra time explaining in detail to the community intensivist the criteria for ECMO so that the next patient they call about is likely a better candidate and they get to hear a "yes." Over time, these calls become shorter and the base of satisfied referrers becomes much wider simply because you took the time to hear them out.

Remote Cannulation

The capability to send a team to another hospital or into the field to remotely cannulate a patient is an exciting prospect, but entails a considerable investment in equipment and demand on the cannulation team. The basic components are contracts with transport systems (ambulance and air), a cannulation team that is on-call (minimum cannulator and perfusionist, first-assist is helpful), and equipment that is packaged in portable form and ready to go. There are innumerable small details that go into making everything operate smoothly on either end of the remote run that are beyond the scope of this chapter. Suffice to say, unless the program director has experience setting up such a program and has secured in advance the resources to do it, it will be difficult to achieve in a freshly started program. However, the benefits of remote cannulation to patient safety and the recognition gained for the cannulating team's hospital are not insignificant, so as a program grows, it is worth considering. Again, seek help and mentorship from an experienced program, and consult ELSO guidelines [10].

eCPR

Similarly, this is an exciting prospect to consider establishing in your hospital, but particularly for a fresh hospital, it is probably the last thing that should be considered. The data remain poor for eCPR outcomes except in very experienced centers, and there is extraordinary opportunity to do more harm than good. eCPR itself is discussed elsewhere in the book, but as a business model, remember that in a young program outcomes are scrutinized and resource utilization is inspected closely. It is also quite easy to swamp your capacity with inappropriate eCPR cases leaving no room for excellent VA-ECMO candidates with higher predicted survival. This is not to say that a structured eCPR program with success is not possible, but it takes an experienced team with highly disciplined criteria and considerable dedication of on-call resources.

Equipment and Disposables

Next to personnel, sourcing equipment can occupy a significant amount of time and effort. There are four categories of equipment that must be secured: large capital expense items (pump consoles, flow meters, heater/coolers), circuit components (pump heads, oxygenators, sensors), cannulas, and then all other specialty materials such as circuit clamps, particular suture, dressings, zip ties, Hoffman clamps, and other items that will be used in the ICU either on a daily basis or during cannulations or circuit exchanges. For all these items, it is the role of the program director and ECMO coordinator to ensure that inventory levels are appropriate and that required items, including backups, are in centralized locations where they can be accessed rapidly. These tasks may also be delegated to perfusionists (common) or specialists.

For many programs, all four categories are sourced from the cardiac ORs and the budgeting falls under the appropriate cardiothoracic surgery or perfusion program. However, as a program grows, sharing equipment may become undesirable as it may compete with OR needs for the same items, or the OR may not want to purchase or store items the ECMO team desires. In this case, purchasing equipment that belongs to the ECMO program or its home ICU makes sense. Cannulas generally are sourced from the same suppliers as the OR, but depending on the preferred cannulation strategy and use of specialty cannulas, there may be opportunity for cheaper bulk purchasing when done through your own cost center. It is the choice of pump and circuit that is the most difficult.

The right choice of pump is, like most everything in an ECMO program's structure, dependent on the needs of the institution. Cost generally is a driving issue, but often benefits also derive from robustness, safety features, and ease of training and use. There are generally two types of systems, nonintegrated and integrated. With nonintegrated systems, the console is bought for the pump head, and the circuit components (pump head and oxygenator) are purchased separately. These systems will generally have a flow sensor but no other included sensors, so any desired pressure transducers or additional flow sensors or bubble detectors would also need to be purchased separately and assembled into the circuit. While this sounds laborious, it is in fact often more economical as these component pieces are the same as used in the OR for bypass cases and are manufactured at scale. Currently, a complete, nonintegrated circuit can be as much as a quarter of the cost of an integrated circuit; however, the integrated circuits' price points are improving as they gain in popularity.

Aside from the need to hand assemble and the resulting greater size of the circuit, the largest drawback to the nonintegrated circuit tends to be its lack of integrated sensors. In general, for simpler patients and experienced providers and specialists, this may not be a problem, but for new programs, programs with complex patients, or programs with higher reliance on non-perfusionist or lesser experienced specialists, having a system with more robust real-time sensors such as drainage pressures, pre- and post-membrane pressures, venous saturations, and bubble detectors may add a layer of safety, simplify circuit maintenance, and reduce training time. They are generally more compact systems as well, making patient transport easier which may be a consideration for programs entertaining remote cannulation and transport.

In the end, almost any system can be made to work with the right balance of ancillary equipment, processes, and training. Whichever primary system is chosen, consider as well a secondary brand to keep available. The advantage of alternate manufacturers is that you have backup in times of manufacturing shortages and also in times of price inflation to flex to another system and leverage pricing. These shortages were real occurrences during COVID in which certain types of oxygenators were just unavailable for a short period. The last option to discuss is that of renting the pump consoles, which is an especially good option for very-low-volume centers or for flexing up during just the peak seasons (e.g., flu season). This can also let you trial a platform without committing the capital expense. Whatever your plans, as you budget, you must budget at least one more pump console that will always be immediately available as a backup in the case of pump failure [5]. In other words, if your planned ECMO capacity is two patients, you would need to own (or lease) three pumps.

Documentation and Charting

There are three general categories of documentation a program needs to maintain. The first is overall documentation on the program itself. This includes written description of all processes, guidelines and protocols including how emergencies are handled, inventory, training guidelines, expectations for all roles in the team, anticoagulation, weaning, consult process, acceptance criteria, etc. Everything that is important to the smooth functioning of the program should be written and readily available to every member of the team as a reference. These documents are also a required part of becoming an ELSO Center of Excellence. Data from patient outcomes and complications, team member training and evaluations, and consult requests and outcomes should also all be gathered, analyzed, documented, and compared against the ECMO team's established guidelines and predetermined goals. This should inform the ongoing revision of the guidelines in the Quality Assurance cycle [5].

The second level of documentation is flow sheet data in the patient's chart. This is accomplished by the bedside specialist at regular intervals (generally every 1–2 h) and includes recording all the current pump parameters (RPM, flows), sensor readings, blood gas results, and possibly hemodynamics if not automatically captured. At the same time, circuit checks are documented including cannula position at the skin, insertion-site integrity, presence of clot in the line, oxygenator or pump, and presence and correct position of any clamps. Histories of alarms or other circuit problems should be both documented and reported to the ECMO team providers. This level of documentation is a standard of care.

The last level of documentation is that of the ECMO team providers. Depending on the country and locality, the documentation requirements for ECMO as a procedure may be different and should be investigated with your local compliance team. However, in general, it is good practice to document the progress of the patient's ECMO run apart from the nonassociated critical care issues. Documenting weaning attempts and other adjustments, complications, current anticoagulation strategy, current setting snapshots, etc. can not only meet documentation requirements for billing purposes but also provide information for later analysis of things like complication rates and timing of weaning that may be useful for program improvement. ECMO providers and the ECMO Program Director should arrive at a common standard for daily documentation of ECMO patients under their care.

Successful Programs

Measures of success for ECMO as a modality are straightforward: Did the patient survive to decannulation and then to discharge? These are easily benchmarked against data from ELSO, and should be regularly. However, these do not alone capture the measure of success for your program, and you should define them as part of your road map. These should become part of your regular review with an aim to improve your program. Some sample measures might include:

1. Number of consults received internally and externally
2. Number of runs per year
3. Complication rates
4. Blood product usage
5. Length of stay
6. Patient family satisfaction
7. Patient follow-up and long-term outcomes
8. Disposable costs and saving opportunities identified
9. Team member retention and satisfaction
10. Team member participation in outside activities (workshops, conferences, etc.)
11. Publications

While it is important to define measures of success for yourself as a program, it is also extremely important to understand what is important to the hospital system and what as a service line you will be held accountable for. These are not always as straightforward as they seem. As an example, an administration may not always be as concerned with poor outcomes if the service is one that is expected by the community and that they do not lose money on and has low impact on other services. Or they may be extremely concerned despite exceedingly good outcomes because the service takes resources such as nursing or space away from other lines. Administrations are always balancing trying to keep many service lines afloat, and it is part of the ECMO program's stewardship to maintain their perception as a service line that is part of that healthy balance. The first step is to understand what is important to your particular hospital:

1. Financial impact (Profitable? Neutral? Loss leader?)
2. Impact on other service lines (OR time, ICU occupancy, nursing ratios, specialist pull from RT/nursing/perfusion)
3. Standard of care or meeting the competition (Is this expected of our level of institution?)

4. Patient outcomes (As compared to national? To local competition? Indexed by acuity?)
5. Prestige and notoriety (Is this something we can market?)

Not all of these are necessarily important to all systems. For instance, many big systems already think that they are as famous and important as they will ever be and will not be moved by appealing to prestige. However, they may care very much that the up and coming competitor has improved outcomes for critically ill patients without worsening length of stay since they started their ECMO program.

That all said, particularly early in a program, what can easily set a program back or even kill it is several back-to-back poor outcomes or long lengths of stay that drain resources. An established program can usually weather this politically with their administration, but new ones do not have a track record to fall back on. For this reason, it is generally advisable early in a program to be very conservative with patient selection criteria. As your program progresses, it may become more aggressive with patient selection, but it is a good idea to continue to benchmark your outcomes, complication rates, and lengths of stay against other ECMO centers in your region with similar characteristics as your hospital and patient population. There are several sources for this data such as the Extracorporeal Life Support Organization (ELSO), commercial quality metric data services, and government health department and ministry statistics. Knowing your own statistics on a regular basis is critical as it is possible to miss worsening performance until your administration brings it to your attention. Generally, this has suboptimal consequences. A good way to provide regular motivation for this data collection is to participate in the ELSO registry, which has the added benefit of giving back to the larger ECMO community [4, 11].

References

1. ELSO guidelines for patient care, respiratory & cardiac support, ECMO in COVID-19: extracorporeal life support organization. Available from: https://www.elso.org/ecmo-resources/elso-ecmo-guidelines.aspx
2. Guerin C, Reignier J, Richard JC, Beuret P, Gacouin A, Boulain T, et al. Prone positioning in severe acute respiratory distress syndrome. N Engl J Med. 2013;368(23):2159–68.
3. Peek GJ, Clemens F, Elbourne D, Firmin R, Hardy P, Hibbert C, et al. CESAR: conventional ventilatory support vs extracorporeal membrane oxygenation for severe adult respiratory failure. BMC Health Serv Res. 2006;6:163.
4. Moll V, Teo EY, Grenda DS, Powell CD, Connor MJ Jr, Gartland BT, et al. Rapid development and implementation of an ECMO program. ASAIO J. 2016;62(3):354–8.
5. Combes A, Brodie D, Bartlett R, Brochard L, Brower R, Conrad S, et al. Position paper for the organization of extracorporeal membrane oxygenation programs for acute respiratory failure in adult patients. Am J Respir Crit Care Med. 2014;190(5):488–96.
6. Turner DA, Williford WL, Peters MA, Thalman JJ, Shearer IR, Walczak RJ Jr, et al. Development of a collaborative program to provide extracorporeal membrane oxygenation for adults with refractory hypoxemia within the framework of a pandemic. Pediatr Crit Care Med. 2011;12(4):426–30.

7. Munoz J, Santa-Teresa P, Tomey MJ, Visedo LC, Keough E, Barrios JC, et al. Extracorporeal membrane oxygenation (ECMO) in adults with acute respiratory distress syndrome (ARDS): a 6-year experience and case-control study. Heart Lung. 2017;46(2):100–5.

8. Jones-Akhtarekhavari J, Tribble TA, Zwischenberger JB. Developing an extracorporeal membrane oxygenation program. Crit Care Clin. 2017;33(4):767–75.

9. Kouch M, Green A, Damuth E, Noel C, Bartock J, Rosenbloom M, et al. Rapid development and deployment of an intensivist-led venovenous extracorporeal membrane oxygenation cannulation program. Crit Care Med. 2022;50(2):e154–e61.

10. Labib A, August E, Agerstrand C, Frenckner B, Laufenberg D, Lavandosky G, et al. Extracorporeal life support organization guideline for transport and retrieval of adult and pediatric patients with ECMO support. ASAIO J. 2022;68(4):447–55.

11. Registry of active ELSO centers using ECMO: extracorporeal life support organization. Available from: https://www.elso.org/registry.aspx

Chapter 3
Indications for ECMO

Suneel Kumar Pooboni

Types of ECMO

There are two basic types of ECMO: venovenous and venoarterial. Venovenous ECMO involves draining the deoxygenated venous blood from a peripheral vein and reinfusion of oxygenated blood into the same vein at a different level or another vein. Venoarterial ECMO implies draining the venous blood from a peripheral vein and reinfusion of oxygenated blood into a systemic artery. In circumstances with inadequate flow or differential flow, additional access lines may have to be secured. These could be venous or arterial. They are labeled as hybrid modes of ECMO.

Patient Selection

ECMO is a useful technology to support heart or lungs in all age groups (neonates, children, and adults) following failure of maximal conventional management. There are two basic criteria to be fulfilled before we consider ECMO:

1. Reversibility of the disease in its natural course
2. No contraindication to limited anticoagulation

In the clinical progression of a disease process, at times, we might not be clear about the reversibility of the disease. Under these circumstances, we support the patient on ECMO while constantly evaluating the degree of reversibility. When it becomes clear that the disease process is irreversible, unless another modality of long-term support such as ventricular assist device (VAD), paracorporeal

S. K. Pooboni (✉)
Department of Pediatric Critical Care, Mediclinic City Hospital, Dubai, UAE

© The Author(s), under exclusive license to Springer Nature Switzerland AG 2024
A. R. Taha et al. (eds.), *ECMO: A Practical Guide to Management*,
https://doi.org/10.1007/978-3-031-59634-6_3

ambulatory lung assist devices, or lung/heart-lung transplantation is available, ECMO support may have to be discontinued after multidisciplinary discussions, including involvement of the family. In these instances, ECMO can be used as a bridge for transplant or similar support. The availability of the definitive modalities of long term varies as per geographical location and access to treatment.

Extracorporeal Life Support Organization (ELSO), as the apex body, has published guidelines for selection of the patients. The primary indication for ECMO is acute severe heart or lung failure or heart failure following failure of maximal conventional measures (ventilation, inotropes, and other measures) with high mortality risk [1]. The extent of lung/heart failure and the mortality risk is measured as precisely as possible using measurements for the appropriate age group and the severity of organ failure.

Optimization of Conventional Measures Prior to ECMO

Failure of maximal conventional ventilation for gas exchange is an indication for considering ECMO support. Generally, patients with ARDS respond reasonably well to advanced methods of critical care, such as various modes of mechanical ventilation with optimal positive end-expiratory pressure (PEEP) and strategies such as permissive hypercapnia, permissive hypoxia, restrictive fluid therapies, diuretic therapies to get rid of cumulative fluid balance including continuous renal replacement therapy (CRRT), positional maneuvers such as proning besides adopting physiotherapy, use of inotropes to help with systemic perfusion, and inhalational pulmonary vasodilators to aid in case of pulmonary hypertension. Though there are selective criteria to help us in assessing the functional capacity of the lungs, the final decision to consider ECMO support depends upon the type of the disease, diagnosis, chances of reversibility, rate of progression of the disease, and the overall experience of the physician. If the referrals take place from a known hospital, it would be ideal to share the ventilatory strategies, medications, and drug infusion policies so that there will not be any confusion while transferring patients across. It helps in the post-ECMO phase as well as in continuing the conventional management after transferring the patient back to the referring hospital.

Ideally, one should consider ECMO support when the risk of mortality reaches 50% and is strongly indicated when mortality risk approaches 80% with conventional therapy [1]. Earlier consideration may be indicated to minimize barotrauma and other morbidities from aggressive conventional therapies [2]. Once the criteria for consideration of ECMO are met, it would be preferable to place the patient on ECMO to minimize lung damage and assist in the recovery process. The longer the ECMO is postponed in eligible patients, the greater are the chances of barotrauma and/or volutrauma.

Justification for ECMO

It is a well-known fact that high-pressure ventilation associated with high ventilatory settings is injurious to the lungs. Ventilator-induced lung injury, a term used synonymously with barotrauma of the lung, is currently viewed as a systemic disease with similar symptoms and macroscopical and microscopical features of experimental acute lung injury, which is not markedly different from the diffuse alveolar damage that is present in human ARDS. It may be associated with conditions such as pulmonary and systemic infections, multisystem organ dysfunction, volutrauma, and barotrauma, resulting in increased morbidity and mortality [2].

Predominantly, ECMO support will be needed under two circumstances:

A. Lung failure
B. Heart failure

Indications/Contraindications

Criteria for the initiation of ECMO include acute pulmonary failure that is potentially reversible and unresponsive to conventional management. Most of the medical conditions which could result in lung failure at various ages present with the following criteria [3]:

- Hypoxemic respiratory failure with a ratio of arterial oxygen tension to fraction of inspired oxygen (PaO_2/FiO_2) of <100 mmHg despite optimization of the ventilator settings, including the tidal volume, positive end-expiratory pressure (PEEP), and inspiratory-to-expiratory (I:E) ratio.

- The Berlin consensus document on acute respiratory distress syndrome (ARDS) suggests ECMO in severe respiratory failure ($PaO_2/FiO_2 < 70$) [4]:
- Hypercapnic respiratory failure (type 2) with an arterial pH less than 7.20 [5]
- Need for ventilatory support as a bridge to lung transplantation following failure of gas exchange

Oxygenation Index

In neonates and children, oxygenation index (OI) has a better relevance in correlating with hypoxia. Differences in clinical practice may influence the diagnosis of hypoxia, especially in the PICU where there is greater variability in ventilator management relative to adult ICUs.

Hypoxemic respiratory failure (HRF) is associated with increased risk of mortality and morbidity and worse neurological outcome. Oxygenation index (OI) is routinely used as an indicator of severity of hypoxemic respiratory failure in neonates, with an arbitrary cutoff of 15 or less for mild HRF, between 16 and 25 for moderate HRF, between 26 and 40 for severe HRF, and more than 40 for very severe HRF [6]. Oxygenation index is calculated as $OI = MAP \times Fio_2 \times 100/Pao_2$, where MAP indicates mean airway pressure and Fio_2 indicates fraction of inspired oxygen [7].

Murray Score

In 1988, Murray and colleagues proposed an expanded definition of ARDS, taking into account various pathophysiological features of the clinical syndrome, which remains as a useful objective indicator of hypoxia in adolescents and adults [8, 9]. The Murray scoring system includes four criteria for the development of ALI/ARDS: a "scoring" of hypoxemia, a "scoring" of respiratory system compliance, chest radiographic findings demonstrating the number of quadrants involved, and level of positive end-expiratory pressure (PEEP). Each criterion receives a score from 0 to 4 according to the severity of the condition. The final score is obtained by dividing the collective score by the number of components that were used. A score of zero indicates no lung injury, a score of 1–2.5 indicates mild to moderate lung injury, and a final score of more than 2.5 indicates the presence of ARDS [10]. A score of more than 3 can be taken as an indication for placement on ECMO.

Murray score for calculation of respiratory failure criteria for ECMO [11]

Parameter score	0	1	2	3	4
PaO_2/FiO_2 (mm Hg)	≥ 300	225–299	175–224	100–174	<100
Chest X-ray (quadrants infiltrated)	Normal	1	2	3	4
PEEP (cm H_2O)	≤ 5	6–8	9–11	12–14	≥ 15
Compliance (ml/cm H_2O)	≥ 80	60–79	40–59	20–39	≤ 19

Source: Putowski, Z.; Szczepańska, A.; Czok, M.; Krzych, Ł.J. V V ECMO in Covid-19—Where Are We Now? Int. J. Environ. Res. Public Health 2021, 18, 1173.https://doi.org/10.3390/ijerph18031173
PaO2 partial pressure of arterial oxygen, *FiO2* fraction of inspired oxygen, *PEEP* positive end-expiratory pressure

Indications as per ELSO Criteria [12]

Murray score of more than 3, P:F ratio of less than 80 on FiO_2 more than 90%.

Indications as per CESAR Trial Criteria [13]

Murray score of more than 3 and potentially reversible respiratory failure.

Indications as per EOLIA Trial Criteria [14]

P/F ratio less than 50, on FiO_2 more than 0.8 for more than 3 h.
P/F ratio less than 80, on FiO_2 more than 0.8 for more than 6 h.
pH less than 7.25 for more than 6 h (respiratory rate increased to 35) adjusted to
keep P $_{plat}$ less than 32.

Venovenous ECMO: Neonates [15]

Indications	Contraindications
Meconium aspiration syndrome	Duration of high-pressure ventilation of more than 7–10 days
Severe respiratory distress syndrome not responding to surfactant	Not able to cope with anticoagulation Prematurity: less than 32 weeks' gestation
Persisting pulmonary hypertension of newborn	Major intraventricular/cerebral bleed (grade 3 or 4 intraventricular hemorrhage)
Severe pneumonias	Established chronic lung disease
Neonatal pertussis	Lethal malformations or congenital anomalies
Congenital diaphragmatic hernia (CDH)	Surfactant protein B deficiency
Multiple pneumothoraces ± bronchopleural fistula	Alveolar capillary dysplasia

Venovenous ECMO: Pediatrics

Indications	Contraindications
Severe pneumonias (viral and bacterial)	Duration of high-pressure ventilation of more than 7–10 days
Acute respiratory distress syndrome (ARDS)	Not able to cope with limited anticoagulation
Refractory status asthmaticus	Major cerebral bleed (grade 3 or 4)
Alveolar lipoproteinosis	
Perioperative support to bronchial (airway) surgery	
Multisystem Inflammatory Syndrome-Children (Unresponsive to conventional measures)	
Air leak syndromes with barotrauma	

Venovenous ECMO: Adults

Indications	Contraindications
ARDS	Acute intracerebral bleed
Pneumonias (viral/bacterial) including COVID, H1N1	Inability to cope with limited anticoagulation
Atypical pneumonia	Severe multiorgan failure
Aspiration syndromes	Duration of high-pressure ventilation of more than 7–10 days
Pulmonary hemorrhage in collagen vascular diseases: vasculitis, Goodpasture syndrome	Advanced age
ARDS: Post-severe contusion of lungs: Post-trauma	Severe multiorgan failure
Near drowning	Preexisting life-limiting disease
Respiratory failure in lung transplant	Irreversibility of organ failure
Bronchopleural fistulas and pulmonary air leaks	
Complex airway management	

Indications for VA-ECMO in Neonates [15]

Indications	Contraindications
Pre-stabilization: Cyanotic congenital heart disease in decompensated shock	Major intraventricular/cerebral bleed (grade 3 or 4 intraventricular hemorrhage)
Resistant arrhythmias in cardiogenic shock	Not able to cope with anticoagulation Prematurity: less than 32 weeks' gestation
Neonatal myocardial infarction	Lethal malformations or congenital anomalies incompatible with life.
Myocarditis	
Postoperative: Inability to come off cardiopulmonary bypass	
Failing heart after cardiac surgery	
ECPR	

Indications for VA-ECMO in Pediatrics

Indications	Contraindications
Extended cardiopulmonary bypass with low cardiac output syndrome	Intracerebral bleed
Myocarditis	Inability to cope with limited anticoagulation
Cardiomyopathy	
Myocardial infarction	
Septic shock	
ECPR	

Indications for VA-ECMO in Adults [16]

Indications	Contraindications
Extended cardiopulmonary bypass with low cardiac output syndrome	Acute intracerebral bleed
Cardiogenic shock: with or without Myocardial Infarction (MI)	Inability to cope with limited anticoagulation
Fulminant myocarditis	Advanced age
Pulmonary hypertension with right-heart failure	
Pulmonary embolus with hemodynamic compromise	
Cardiac arrest (assisted CPR)	
Poisoning with medications (overdose)	
Sepsis-induced cardiomyopathy	
Bridge to decision for transplant or VAD (LVAD/ BiVAD)	
ECPR	
Inability to come off cardio-pulmonary bypass	
Low cardiac Syndrome Post-cardiac surgery	
Severe Septic (vaso-dilatory) shock	

Indications for Central Cannulation

If the patient can't come off Cardio Pulmonary bypass post-cardiac surgery, it is possible to place the patient on ECMO support by resorting to central cannulation (Fig. 3.1). As per the improvement in cardiac condition, the decision to decannulate or convert to peripheral ECMO can be considered after 48 to 72 hours. Central cannulation is also recommended in septic shock needing high cardiac output as well as to treat those in vasodilatory shock. In central cannulation, the placement of cannulas will be in a chamber of the heart or the proximal vena cava through a median sternotomy incision or related surgical technique. In this case, the common postcardiotomy configuration for venoarterial support with right atrial drainage, a left atrial vent, and aortic return would be "RAva-AO." Left-sided support with drainage from the left ventricle and aortic return would be "LV-AO," and right-sided support from the right atrium to the pulmonary artery would be "RA-PA" [17]. The risks of bleeding, infection, and injury to vessels are greater compared to peripheral cannulation. The advantage of this technique is that it can provide the best perfusion flow and off-load the left ventricle.

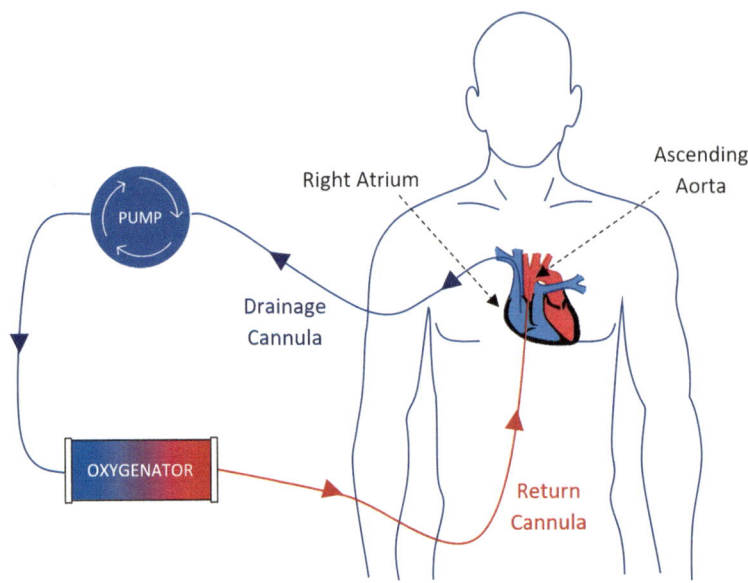

Fig. 3.1 "Illustration of central ECMO cannulation"

VV Versus VA Versus VAV

Advantages and Disadvantages with Hybrid Modes

So far, hybrid ECMO configurations represented a minority of ECMO cannulation modifications in actual practice. The frequency of hybrid configurations is increasing in some practices to 10–15% as we come to better understanding of disease pathophysiology and adaptation of different combinations of cannulas to drain/perfuse different chambers. In addition to traditional ECMO cannulation, changes in the condition of the patient or the occurrence of specific complications (i.e., differential hypoxia, cerebral hypoxia, or left ventricular dilation) may require modifications in cannulation strategies or the combination of ECMO with additional invasive or minimally invasive procedures, to improve organ function and ECMO efficiency. These are called as "hybrid" strategies, such as the addition of a third or fourth ECMO cannula to improve venous drainage and/or optimize systemic hemodynamics/oxygenation, or the implementation of surgical or percutaneous unloading of the left ventricle (LV), to reduce dilation of cardiac chambers and pulmonary edema [18].

Hybrid ECMO might also include addition of another device such as intra-aortic balloon pump, Impella, and others; insertion of drainage cannula into pulmonary artery as an alternative to manage refractory hypoxemia and right ventricular dysfunction; using double pumps to regulate the flows in case of Harlequin syndrome; and other modifications. It is an evolving science.

VV to VVV Configuration If the systemic hypoxia persists despite optimizing fluid volume and after excluding recirculation, improving the amount of blood flow through the oxygenator might help the situation. We can achieve additional flow by inserting additional venous drainage cannula and connecting it via Y connection (Fig. 3.2).

VV to VAV Configuration Let us think about using femoral vein for drainage and internal jugular return for respiratory failure (ARDS). If this patient develops right-heart failure or left-heart failure or biventricular failure, returning part of the oxygenated blood to the femoral artery will help in off-loading the heart (Fig. 3.3).

Fig. 3.2 VV to VVV
ECMO cannulation

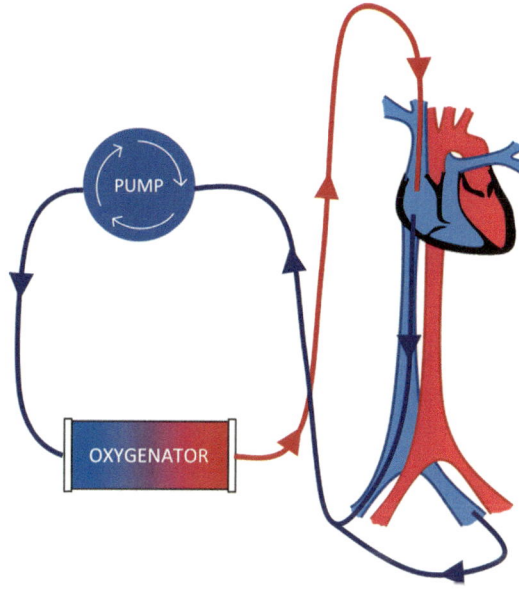

Fig. 3.3 VV to VAV
configuration

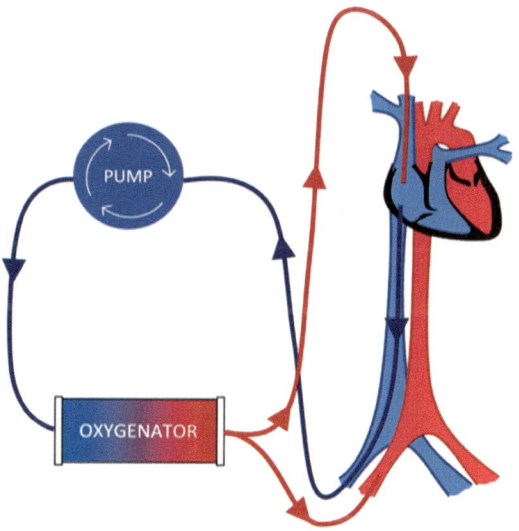

Fig. 3.4 VA to VVA configuration

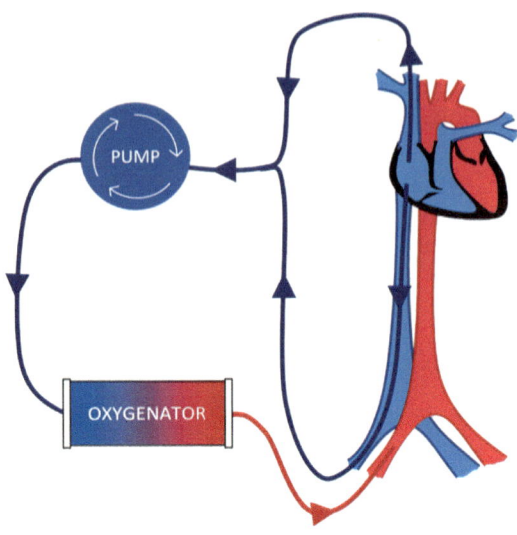

By doing this, we are providing additional cardiac support to the respiratory support.

VA to VVA Configuration In traditional VA cannulation using femoral vein for drainage and femoral artery for return, for off-loading the heart, secondary drainage cannula can be inserted into internal jugular vein (Fig. 3.4).

VA to VAV Configuration In peripheral VA ECMO with severe lung dysfunction, once the heart starts to eject deoxygenated blood, it results in differential hypoxia (Harlequin syndrome) with cerebral anoxia. Provision of oxygenated blood by an additional cannula into jugular vein resolves the situation. In this configuration, one is a drainage cannula and the other two are return cannulas (Fig. 3.5).

In the nomenclature of hybrid cannulation, in the venovenous setup, for example in VV or VVV configuration, the last V always represents return line. To the contrary, in VA, VVA, VAV, etc. configurations, as we know, A represents return line and the V after A also represents additional return line. In other words, V preceding A represents drainage line, while V after A represents return line.

In hybrid cannulation, monitoring the flow on the return cannula with flow sensors and regulating the flow selectively with the help of occlude devices are essential. Uncorrected differential flow might result in ECMO output failure and even death. Hence, for the beginners, hybrid cannulation and flow management should not be taken easily. It needs understanding and practice.

Fig. 3.5 VA to VAV
configuration

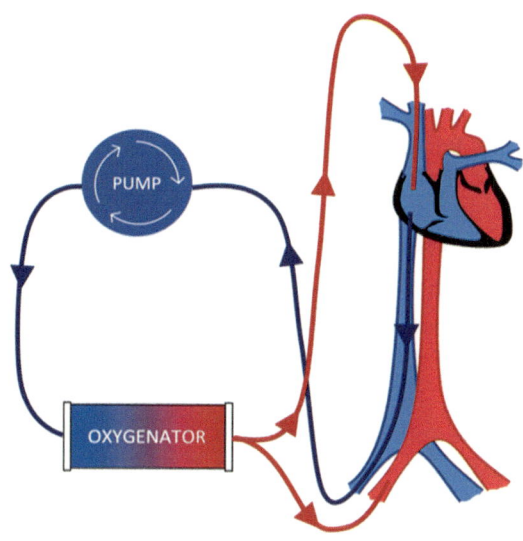

Special Groups

Pregnancy Acute respiratory failure in pregnancy can be treated with ECMO for cases of ARDS following failure of conventional management. Certain special positions have to be tried for safe cannulation in view of the gravid uterus pressing on the blood vessels. ECMO has been used successfully as a salvage therapy during pregnancy and the postpartum period.

Malignancy If the underlying malignancy has good prognosis and chances of cure, ECMO can be considered, e.g., childhood leukemia. Praveena et al. quoted in their paper that reports from 2014 to 2019 have particularly implied that patients with hematological malignancies requiring ECMO have an increasingly favorable prognosis, some even exhibiting long-term survival. However, this data consists of small retrospective studies and case reports. Retrospective studies revealed long-term disease-free survival, particularly when ECMO served as a bridge through chemotherapy [19].

Transplant: Pre and Post
Indications:
    Donor: to extend the quality of donor organs:

To keep the perfusion and homeostasis in the brain-dead donor
Extracorporeal interval support for organ retrieval (EISOR)

Recipient:

- Pretransplant: for stabilization
- Posttransplant:

  - Primary graft dysfunction
  - Graft rejection

ELECMO ECMO for elective high-risk procedures:

High-risk, complex tracheal surgeries
Complex tracheal/bronchial repairs
Complex bronchopulmonary lavage

High-risk cardiac procedures such as left main coronary arterial stenting, ablation of refractory ventricular arrhythmias, rapid-access bedside thermotherapy (RABT), or extracorporeal warming in case of cold-water drowning.

Triage and Limited Resources

Venovenous extracorporeal membrane oxygenation (VV-ECMO), a resource-intensive approach to managing severe respiratory failure, was utilized to treat severe ARDS resulting from COVID with high mortality in the initial part of 2020. With experience building up over the next few months, the survival figures improved. However, as it was the pandemic period, it was expected that the candidacy of patients should follow the same pre-pandemic rules, taking into account the severity of the acute disease, the burden of any eventual comorbidity, and the chances of a good quality of life after recovery, but the current capacity of the healthcare system should also be considered, and frequently reassessed, with varying implications in countries with wide geographic and healthcare variations [20]. SWAAC ELSO member countries have a variable healthcare provision system too. In some countries, ECMO provision for deserving cases (from disease severity) will be looked after by the governments themselves, whereas in other countries, it remained predominantly a treatment modality available to higher socio-economic classes as per the affordability.

Ethical and legal aspects pertinent to the triage of this resource-intensive, but potentially lifesaving, therapy in the setting of the COVID-19 pandemic were evaluated at different time points in the pandemic period. Given considerations relevant to VV-ECMO use, additional emphasis has been placed on emerging hospital resource scarcity and disproportionate representation of healthcare workers among the ill [21].

It is a well-known fact that the availability of ICU beds and ECMO machines widely varies around the world. In critical conditions, such as a global pandemic, the establishment of contingency capacity tiers might help in defining to which conditions and subjects ECMO can be offered. In the initial guidance document published by ELSO in April 2020, they mentioned that the decision to put a patient on ECMO should be a local (hospital and regional) responsibility. It is a case-by-case decision that should be reassessed regularly based on the overall patient load, staffing, and other resource constraints, as well as local governmental, regulatory, or hospital policies. If the hospital must commit all resources to other patients, then ECMO should not be considered until the resources stabilize. If the hospital feels that ECMO can be safely provided, then it should be offered to patients with a good prognosis with the use of ECMO and perhaps to other patients who qualify for ECMO support. Use of ECMO in patients with a combination of advanced age, multiple comorbidities, or multiple-organ failure should be rare [22]. A frequent reassessment of the resource saturation, possibly integrated within a regional health-care coordination system (in countries where such system exists), may be of help to triage the patients who most likely will benefit from advanced techniques, especially when capacities are limited.

Consent and Family Preparation

Obtaining consent/assent for ECMO is a complex process. In the vast majority of instances, informed consent cannot be obtained from the critically ill patient on the ventilator or his/her family members. The obstacles to obtaining informed consent are multiple and include some of the following:

(a) Unconscious patient on sedatives
(b) Understanding of the family members about ECMO
(c) Critical time pressures
(d) Complexity of disease process and varying outcomes
(e) Financial limitations/health insurance coverage as the case may be
(f) Influence of extended family members, friends of the family, or next of kin
(g) Trusting as an expert recommendation

The informed consent process is an exercise of a person's autonomy. As physicians, we are supposed to explain the intervention we are planning, with detailed explanation about the process, advantages, disadvantages, and uncertainties, eliciting patient/carer's understanding. It is understandable that emotion and intellect have an enormous impact on the process of informed consent and its outcome.

The difficulty in carrying out the informed consent process while suggesting ECMO as the treatment option is the time pressure. When patients are in cardiac arrest or circulatory collapse, for practical reasons, they are dead. Those patients cannot be educated about either their condition or their options for treatment. In most instances, consent is assumed.

If ECMO is planned for a deteriorating patient already on maximal conventional management, more time may be available for a consent discussion—in most instances, the patient, usually sedated on the ventilator to the point of incompetence to give consent—but the next of kin (family) is still likely to sense both urgency and a lack of alternatives to arrive at the decision-making.

It is understandable that patients/family may not be aware that, at the simplest level, consent for ECMO entails consent for the insertion of at least one large-bore venous cannula and most often a large-bore arterial cannula. Consent for ECMO in the setting of cardiac arrest is implicit consent for all of the associated life support measures, which include intubation and mechanical ventilation, inotropic support, and often renal replacement therapy. As the clinical course of the patient varies, the extent of supportive services needed may vary from time to time. Onset of nosocomial infections might alter the outcome.

Extracorporeal life support therapies are generally called upon in the context of severe, life-threatening conditions usually after maximizing other options to support life, and the initial decision to use them is frequently emergent and does not allow for a robust informed consent discussion. Informed consent for ECLS is not realistically possible; the ethical implications of this fact should be taken into account as its use becomes yet more widespread [23].

As per the ELSO guidance, the cannulation consent process should explicitly involve discontinuation of ECMO care if ECMO is actively harming the patient (e.g., severe intracerebral bleeding or clotting). In different countries, the practice is likely to be variable, respecting local laws, as per the guidance of the ethics committee.

Despite these limitations, taking informed consent is crucial before putting any patient on ECMO. The physician, most conversant with the ECMO, should explain the family about the procedure, its need, risks and benefits, and outcomes keeping in prospect of the clinical condition of the patient. It would be ideal to quote outcomes from their own experience. We should give family time to think about the procedure and come back for further clarifications. With the guidance, each institution should frame their consent form. Regular briefings about the patient's condition should be conducted throughout the hospital stay.

COVID and ECMO

The COVID pandemic caused by coronavirus-19 left devastating effects on the world's population. The mortality rate to a viral infection, unknown to the mankind before, left the world with much suffering. We are still in the process of understanding the long-term effects of the COVID. The rehabilitation process following recovery from severe COVID might extend to several months.

In the initial period following the onset of COVID in 2020, ELSO recommended ECMO in the institutions where it is done regularly as universal healthcare takes precedence to high-cost treatments such as ECMO. Observations and learning from the ground level made us understood the emergence of new centers during the time of need and performing reasonably well [10]. No doubt, COVID led to financial difficulties in many households in the developing world.

ECMO is a helpful therapy in severe ARDS secondary to COVID-19 infection like other viral infections. ELSO provided the medical community with guidelines and constant updates on its website as a resource for centers which may be called on to manage COVID-19 patients. For real-time updates, information was shared on ELSO's social media accounts at Twitter (@ELSOOrg and @ECMOed) and Facebook (https://www.facebook.com/ELSO.Org) as well as the ECMOed COVID-19 page (https://elso.blog/category/2019ncov-2/) [24].

At the time of the initial breakout of the pandemic, ELSO published its guidance about the consideration of ECMO for COVID-19 patients as "this decision is a local (hospital and regional) responsibility. It is a case-by-case decision that should be reassessed regularly based on the overall patient load, staffing, and other resource constraints, as well as local governmental, regulatory, or hospital policies. If the hospital must commit all resources to other patients, then ECMO should not be considered until the resources stabilize. If the hospital feels that ECMO can be safely provided, then it should be offered to patients with a good prognosis with the use of ECMO and perhaps to other patients who qualify for ECMO support" [25].

In 2021, ELSO updated guidelines for the management of COVID-19 ECMO [26].

The great majority of COVID-19 patients (>90%) requiring ECMO were supported using venovenous (VV) ECMO for acute respiratory distress syndrome (ARDS). While COVID-19 ECMO-run duration may be longer than in non-COVID-19 ECMO patients, published mortality appears to be similar between the two groups. Conventional two-site (VA and VV) and multisite, e.g., veno-arteriovenous (VAV), cannulation strategies, as well as VV dual-lumen cannulas, as needed to address the underlying problems, are appropriate for use in patients with COVID-19. There are no data to suggest deviation from conventional ECMO device or patient management when applying ECMO for COVID-19 patients. Rarely, children may require ECMO support for COVID-19-related ARDS, myocarditis, or multisystem inflammatory syndrome in children (MIS-C); conventional selection criteria and management practices should be the standard (Figs. 3.6 and 3.7).

COVID-19 cases in the ELSO registry (as per the information in May 2024)

Total COVID 19 Confirmed cases on ECMO	Patients who initiated ECMO at least 90 days ago COVID-19 Confirmed	COVID-19 In-hospital Mortality
17,720	16,290	48%

Source: COVID-19 registry dashboard: https://www.elso.org/ (accessed on 27th May 2024)

These figures do not include the cases that were not reported to the ELSO. It is estimated that the total number of cases of COVID-19 treated on ECMO for ARDS in developing countries would be much higher.

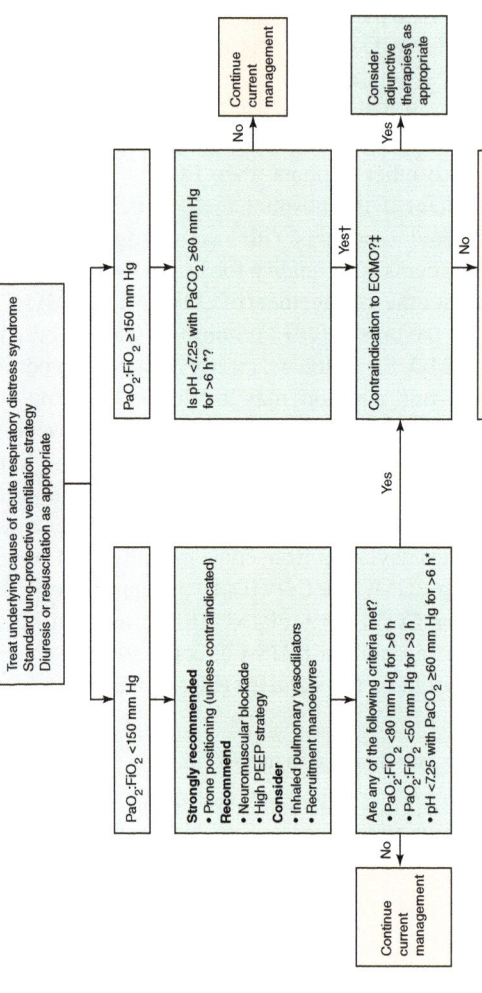

Fig. 3.6 Algorithm for the management of acute respiratory distress syndrome, including indications for ECMO. (Reproduced from Extracorporeal Membrane Oxygenation for COVID-19: Updated 2021 Guidelines from the Extracorporeal Life Support Organization ASAIO J. 2021 May 1;67 (5):485–495. doi: 10.1097/MAT.0000000000001422. Reproduced with permission from Christine Stead, ELSO)

Algorithm for the management of acute respiratory distress syndrome, including indications for ECMO. *With respiratory rate increased to 35 breaths per minute and mechanical ventilation settings adjusted to keep a plateau airway pressure of <32 cm H₂O. +Consider neuromuscular blockade. ‡There are no absolute contraindications that are agreed upon except end-stage respiratory failure when lung transplantation will not be considered; exclusion used in the EOLIA trial can be taken as a conservative approach to CMO contraindications. For example, neuromuscular blockade, high PEEP strategy, inhaled pulmonary vasodilators, recruitment maneuvers, and high-frequency oscillatory ventilation. ¶ Recommend early ECMO as per EOLIA trial criteria; salvage CMO, which involves deferral of CMO initiation until further decompensation (as in the crossovers to ECMO in the EOLIA control group), is not supported by the evidence but might be preferable to not initiating ECMO at all in such patients. Credit: Abrams et al. ECMO, extracorporeal membrane oxygenation; EOLIA, Extracorporeal Membrane Oxygenation to Rescue Lung Injury in Severe Acute Respiratory Distress Syndrome; PaCO2, partial pressure of carbon dioxide in arterial blood; PaO₂:FiO₂, ratio of partial pressure of oxygen in arterial blood to the fractional concentration of oxygen in inspired air; PEEP, positive end-expiratory pressure

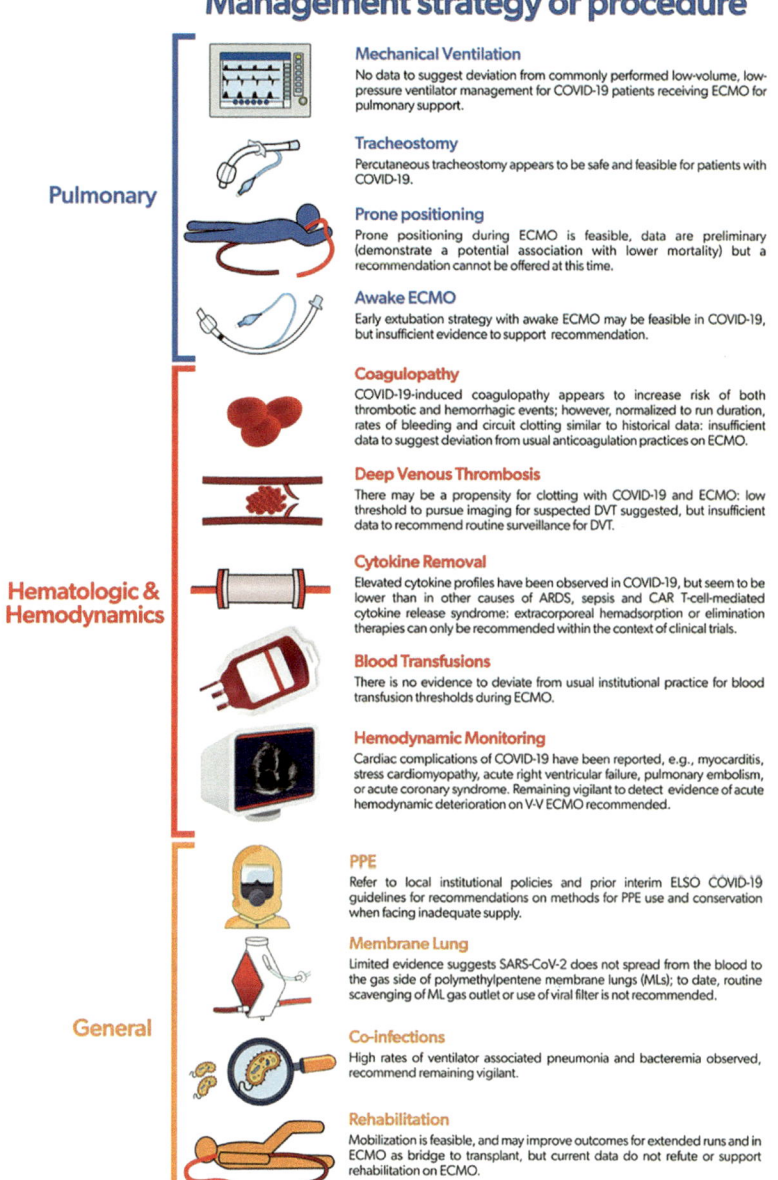

Fig. 3.7 Recommendations for ongoing care and rehabilitation for patients with COVID-19 receiving ECMO. *ARDS* acute respiratory distress syndrome, *CAR* chimeric antigen receptor, *COVID-19* coronavirus disease 2019, *DVT* deep venous thrombosis, *ECMO* extracorporeal membrane oxygenation, *ELSO* Extracorporeal Life Support Organization, *ML* membrane lung, *PPE* personal protective equipment, *SARS-CoV-2* severe acute respiratory syndrome coronavirus-2, *VV* venovenous. (Reproduced from Extracorporeal Membrane Oxygenation for COVID-19: Updated 2021 Guidelines from the Extracorporeal Life Support Organization ASAIO J. 2021 May 1;67 (5):485–495. doi: 10.1097/MAT.0000000000001422. Reproduced with kind courtesy of Christine Stead, ELSO, with permission)

Recommendations Specific to COVID-19

Since COVID-19 patients may be associated with a hypercoagulable state, it is advisable to consider targeting anticoagulation at the higher end of normal ECMO parameters [27].

- Limited evidence suggests that SARS-CoV-2 does not pass from the blood to the gas side of polymethyl pentane oxygenator membrane. Use of viral filters for routine scavenging of gas exiting the membrane oxygenator is not recommended.
- Anticoagulation should be maintained when using lower ECMO blood flow rates (<2 L in adults) given the greater risk of circuit thrombosis in COVID-19 ECMOs.
- Patients with a hypercoagulable status may benefit from antiplatelet agents (such as aspirin, clopidogrel, prasugrel, ticagrelor), but there is insufficient data to recommend. Both thrombocytopenia and prothrombotic states have been reported in patients with COVID-19 [24].
- Patients with COVID-19 may have secondary hemophagocytic lymphohistiocytosis [28].
- If there is any clinical suspicion, screening should be performed and hematologist can be consulted.

For lung failure, futility of a prolonged run should be established on a case-by-case basis.

If lung transplantation is available, the team should be involved for evaluation at the right time.

In cases of cardiac failure, meaningful recovery of heart usually occurs on ECMO by days 5–7. If there are no chances of recovery by this time, it has to be considered futile, and transition to a long-term support should be considered (VAD or transplant).

The subsequent variants of COVID-19 following delta strain, such as Omicron, BA.1, BA.2, BA.3, BA.4, BA.5, and descendent lineages, are not severe as the previous variants. Vaccination might have partly helped in building the immunity. As the COVID-19 presentation is milder nowadays, ARDS and need for ECMO are also less common.

References

1. https://www.elso.org/ecmo-resources/elso-ecmo-guidelines.aspx
2. Lewandowski K. Extracorporeal membrane oxygenation for severe acute respiratory failure. Crit Care. 2000;4(3):156–68.
3. https://www.uptodate.com/contents/extracorporeal-membrane-oxygenation-ecmo-in-adults. Accessed 26 Oct 2022.
4. Ferguson ND, Fan E, Camporota L, et al. The Berlin definition of ARDS: an expanded rationale, justification, and supplementary material. Intensive Care Med. 2012;38:1573.

5. Braune S, Sieweke A, Brettner F, et al. The feasibility and safety of extracorporeal carbon dioxide removal to avoid intubation in patients with COPD unresponsive to noninvasive ventilation for acute hypercapnic respiratory failure (ECLAIR study): multicentre case-control study. Intensive Care Med. 2016;42:1437.
6. Walsh-Sukys MC, Bauer RE, Cornell DJ, Friedman HG, Stork EK, Hack M. Severe respiratory failure in neonates: mortality and morbidity rates and neurodevelopmental outcomes. J Pediatr. 1994;125(1):104–10. https://doi.org/10.1016/S0022-3476(94)70134-2.
7. Golombek SG, Young JN. Efficacy of inhaled nitric oxide for hypoxic respiratory failure in term and late preterm infants by baseline severity of illness: a pooled analysis of three clinical trials. Clin Ther. 2010;32(5):939–48. https://doi.org/10.1016/j.clinthera.2010.04.023.
8. Murray JF, Matthay MA, Luce JM, Flick MR. An expanded definition of the adult respiratory distress syndrome. Am Rev Respir Dis. 1988;138:720–3.
9. Raghavendran K, Napolitano LM. ALI and ARDS: challenges and advances. Crit Care Clin. 2011;27(3):429–37. https://doi.org/10.1016/j.ccc.2011.05.006.
10. Rabie AA, Azzam MH, Al-Fares AA, Abdelbary A, Mufti HN, Hassan IF, Chakraborty A, Oza P, Elhazmi A, Alfoudri H, Pooboni SK, Al Harthy A, Brodie D, Combes A, Zakhary B, Shekar K, Antonini MV, Barrett NA, Peek G, Arabi YM. Extracorporeal membrane oxygenation in the Middle East and India during the COVID-19 pandemic. Intensive Care Med. 2021;47(8):887–95.
11. Putowski Z, Szczepańska A, Czok M, Krzych ŁJ. Veno-venous extracorporeal membrane oxygenation in Covid-19 – where are we now? Int J Environ Res Public Health. 2021;18:1173. https://doi.org/10.3390/ijerph18031173.
12. ELSO guidelines for cardiopulmonary extracorporeal life support. 2017.
13. Peek GJ, Mugford M, Tiruvoipati R, et al. Efficacy and economic assessment of conventional ventilatory support versus extracorporeal membrane oxygenation for severe adult respiratory failure (CESAR): a multicentre randomised controlled trial. Lancet. 2009;374(9698):1351–63. https://doi.org/10.1016/S0140-6736(09)61069-2.
14. Combes A, Hajage D, Capellier G, Demoule A, et al. EOLIA Trial Group, REVA, and ECMONet. Extracorporeal Membrane Oxygenation for Severe Acute Respiratory Distress Syndrome. N Engl J Med. 2018;378(21):1965–75. https://doi.org/10.1056/NEJMoa1800385. PMID: 29791822.
15. Pooboni SK. Neonatal extra corporeal membrane oxygenation. Indian J Thorac Cardiovasc Surg. 2021;37(4):411–20.
16. Mehta H, Eisen HJ, Cleveland JC Jr. Indications and complications for VA-ECMO for cardiac failure. Expert analysis. J Am Coll Cardiol. 2015. Published online 14th July 2015. accessed on 29th May 2024.
17. Conrad SA, Broman LM, Taccone FS, Lorusso BRH, et al. The Extracorporeal Life Support Organization Maastricht Treaty for nomenclature in extracorporeal life support. A position paper of the extracorporeal life support organization. Am J Respir Crit Care Med. 2018;198(4):447–51. https://doi.org/10.1164/rccm.201710-2130cp.
18. Brasseur A, Scolletta S, Lorusso R, Taccone F. Hybrid extracorporeal membrane oxygenation. J Thorac Dis. 2018, 10(Suppl 5):S707–15. https://doi.org/10.21037/jtd.2018.03.84.
19. Tathineni P, Pandya M, Chaar B. The utility of extracorporeal membrane oxygenation in patients with hematologic malignancies: a literature review. Cureus. 2020;12(7):e9118. Published online 2020 Jul 10. https://doi.org/10.7759/cureus.9118.
20. Nardelli P, Scandroglio AM, De Piero ME, Mariani S, Lorusso R. Selection criteria and triage in extracorporeal membrane oxygenation during coronavirus disease 2019. Review. Curr Opin Crit Care. 2022;28(6):674–80. https://doi.org/10.1097/MCC.0000000000000998.
21. Murugappan KR, Walsh DP, Mittel A, Sontag D, Shaefia S. Veno-venous extracorporeal membrane oxygenation allocation in the COVID-19 pandemic. J Crit Care. 2021;61:221–6. Published online 2020 Nov 13. https://doi.org/10.1016/j.jcrc.2020.11.004.
22. Bartlett RH, Ogino MT, Brodie D, McMullan DM, Lorusso R, MacLaren G, Stead CM, Rycus P, et al. Initial ELSO guidance document: ECMO for COVID-19 patients with severe car-

diopulmonary failure. ASAIO J. 2020;66(5):472–4. Published online 2020 Apr 1. https://doi.org/10.1097/MAT.0000000000001173.

23. Peetz AB, Sadovnikoff N, O'Connor MF. Is informed consent for extracorporeal life support even possible? AMA J Ethics. 2015;17(3):236–42.
24. https://www.elso.org/covid19. Accessed 29 Oct 2022.
25. https://www.elso.org/Portals/0/Files/pdf/ECMO%20for%20COVID%2019%20 Guidance%20Document.Final%2003.24.2020.pdf. Accessed 29 Oct 2022.
26. Badulak J, Antonini V, Stead C, Shekerdemian L, Paden M, Bartlett R, et al. ELSO COVID-19 Working Group Members; Extracorporeal Membrane Oxygenation for COVID-19: updated 2021 guidelines from the Extracorporeal Life Support Organization. ASAIO J. 2021;67(5):485–95. https://doi.org/10.1097/MAT.0000000000001422.
27. Klok FA, Kruip MJHA, van der Meer NJM, et al. Incidence of thrombotic complications in critically ill ICU patients with COVID-19. Thromb Res. 2020;191:145–7.
28. Mehta P, McAuley DF, Brown M, Sanchez E, Tattersall RS, Manson JJ. COVID-19: consider cytokine storm syndromes and immunosuppression. Lancet. 2020;395(10229):1033–4.

Chapter 4
Physics and Technology

Alain Lamontagne and Casey Frost Miller

Many adaptations and modifications have been created using artificial lung technology since the mid-twentieth century, beginning with the very first Gibbon-screen oxygenator used in 1955 during the first series of open-heart procedures (reference pg 11, Gravlee) to the helix reservoir bubble oxygenator, rotating disk oxygenator, silicone oxygenator, hollow-fiber membrane oxygenator, and polymethyl pentene (PMP) oxygenator. PMP oxygenators have been the gold standard choice for extracorporeal life support (ECLS)/extracorporeal membrane oxygenation (ECMO) due to its longevity threshold, lower priming volume, decreased blood path resistance, and improved gas exchange than its predecessor, the silicone membrane oxygenator [2]. Historically, external heat exchangers for ECMO were located distal to the oxygenator. The addition of an integrated heat exchanger in the PMP allows for more effective control of patient core temperature management. Patients may have increased incidence of accidental hypothermia due to extracorporeal blood in tubing, membrane lung, and other circuit components. Total circuit volume can be upwards of 600 ml of blood with indirect contact with cool ambient air; therefore, temperature management is necessary with this patient population.

The ability of a modern-day oxygenator must be able to mimic the capabilities of a native lung. Total surface area for an artificial lung is <5% of that of a native lung; therefore, external pressures (medical grade air, oxygen) must work at higher pressures to compensate for lessened gas exchange surface. In normal pulmonary vasculature, red blood cells pass through pulmonary capillaries in a single-file manner; this creates less distance for oxygen diffusion with an increase in oxygen transfer.

A. Lamontagne
Department of Perfusion Services, Emory Healthcare, Atlanta, GA, USA
e-mail: alain.lamontagne@emoryhealthcare.org

C. F. Miller (✉)
Department of Cardiothoracic Surgery, Emory University Hospital, Atlanta, GA, USA
e-mail: casey.miller@emoryhealthcare.org

Maximum oxygen transfer at standard temperature and pressure for a membrane lung can be upwards of 400–600 mL/min, respectively. However, a native lung can produce 2000 mL/min of oxygen transfer. Ultimately, increased surface area, decreased blood path width/length, and membrane thickness grant the native lung to be superior.

Blood Flow

Blood draining from a cannula placed in a large vein will drain kinetically into the associated pump tethered to the ECMO circuit. The pump head (centrifugal or roller pump) must always be configured proximally to the oxygenator with regard to the blood path. Blood flows continuously through the oxygenator beginning at the inlet port and passes through the oxygenator and around the hollow fibers necessary for gas exchange; oxygenated blood then exits the oxygenator and is propelled back into the patient via artery or vein.

Gas flow travels through porous hollow fibers of the membrane oxygenator and then diffuses into regional blood. The rate of gas exchange is determined by the partial pressure difference between gas and blood. In a normally functioning oxygenator, $PaCO_2$ values will foster an indirect relationship to gas flow. Blood flow must continuously flow through the oxygenator to participate in gas exchange. Stagnant blood, as when the ECMO tubing is clamped and flow is disrupted, cannot participate in gas exchange.

Blood can be warmed or cooled by utilizing an external water source that can be attached directly to the oxygenator. Specific examples include the Quadrox CardioHelp system. Water is passed through a separate set of polypropylene fibers, which regulates blood temperature as it passes through the oxygenator; this occurs without any communication between the water and blood [3]. It is generally recommended to utilize this to maintain normothermia and avoid complications associated with temperature dysregulation.

Centrifugal Pumps

Centrifugal pumps, as often used in extracorporeal life support (ECLS), are afterload-dependent and nonocclusive pumps. Design of centrifugal pumps can vary and may include cone or a vaned impeller [i.e., the centerpiece of the pump, cased in a plastic housing, which spins and propels blood forward when rotating rapidly at an increased revolution per minute (RPM)]. RPM alone will not generate a constant flow. Any restriction or resistance downstream [i.e., vascular resistance, cannula size (inner diameter), malposition of the cannula, kinked tubing, or obstruction] may inhibit flow delivered to the patient. Centrifugal pumps require a flow meter/ultrasonic flow probe to quantify pump flow. Increases in resistance distal to the pump will be indirectly related to systemic pump flow. Due to the nonocclusive characteristics of centrifugal pumps, when circuitry is connected to a patient's systemic vasculature, retrograde flow back through the pump head will occur if zero RPM is being generated. Thus, patient systemic pressures could drop drastically as native blood flow is being diverted through the cannula placed in a large vessel, back down through the pump, causing exsanguination or air being aspirated into the arterial line via purse-string sutures. To avoid this potential error, it is important to keep the pump head at phlebostatic axis to prevent gravity drainage in the event RPM returns to zero. It is also important to ensure that the arterial line is always clamped when the pump head is not running to prevent catastrophic complications.

A desirable advantage to centrifugal pumps is the considerable decrease in propensity to deliver a massive air embolism. This is because 40–50 mL of entrained air will de-prime the pump head and will stop pumping (note: numerous smaller, yet equally harmful, microbubbles can still be passed and delivered to the patient). Centrifugal pumps will not generate as much negative pressure on the inlet side as a roller pump will. Therefore, cavitation is significantly less likely when using a centrifugal pump.

Sensors and Safety Components

As technology for ECLS evolves, sensors and safety components are becoming more readily available. While some systems only offer the ability to monitor pump rotations per minute (RPMs) and flow derived in liters per minute, other systems provide advanced monitoring of pre- and post-membrane pressures, temperature, oxygen content of blood returning to the oxygenator, and estimates of patient hemoglobin. These circuits have sensors that allow close monitoring of device perimeters to notify clinicians of possible impending complications.

Safety components for consoles may also provide audible alarms for preset safety settings [1]. Alarms can be set for early recognition of even slight changes for the patient or the circuit. These systems may also possess sensors that detect air bubbles entrained in the circuit and may prevent forward flow in the event air is detected. The incorporation of sensors and safety components assists in reducing the risks associated with ECLS care for patients.

EMR Integration

Along similar lines, many new products are emerging to assist with the integration of ECLS data into the electronic medical record (EMR). The third-party products assist with transcribing pertinent ECLS data into the EMR in efforts to decrease potential errors from manual entry. Many of these products also allow remote clinician monitoring.

References

1. ELSO. ECMO extracorporeal cardiopulmonary support in critical care. 5th ed. The Red Book; 2017.
2. Khoshbin E, et al. Poly-methyl pentene oxygenators have improved gas exchange capability and reduced transfusion requirements in adult extracorporeal membrane oxygenation. ASAIO J. 2005;51(3):281–7. https://doi.org/10.1097/01.mat.0000159741.33681.f1.
3. Maul T, Nelson J, Wearden P. Paracorporeal lung devices: thinking outside the box. Front Pediatr. 2018;6:243. https://doi.org/10.3389/fped.2018.00243.

Chapter 5
Physiology I: Venovenous ECMO

María Martínez Martínez ⓘ

Venovenous ECMO (VV-ECMO) injects oxygenated blood in the venous circulation and provides support to the failing lungs. The aim of this chapter is to review respiratory physiology, determinants of oxygen transport, and basic management of VV-ECMO support.

Respiratory Physiology

The respiratory system facilitates gas exchange, vital for cellular metabolism and function. Oxygen (O_2) and carbon dioxide (CO_2) passively diffuse through the alveolocapillary membrane in the lungs. Oxygen is transported through the blood to the capillaries, where it is extracted and utilized. CO_2 is a byproduct of the cellular metabolism and is gathered in the capillaries and exhaled through the lungs.

Respiratory insufficiency develops when the lungs are unable to oxygenate and/or decarboxylate the blood. The physiologic mechanisms of respiratory insufficiency are hypoventilation, diffusion alteration, shunt, and alteration of the ventilation-perfusion relationship.

M. Martínez (✉)
Intensive Care Medicine Department - ECMO Team, Hospital Universitari Vall d'Hebron, Barcelona, Spain

SODIR Research Group, Vall d'Hebron Institut de Recerca, Barcelona, Spain
e-mail: maria.martinez@vallhebron.cat

© The Author(s), under exclusive license to Springer Nature Switzerland AG 2024
A. R. Taha et al. (eds.), *ECMO: A Practical Guide to Management*,
https://doi.org/10.1007/978-3-031-59634-6_5

Ventilation, Diffusion, and Perfusion

Blood oxygenation and decarboxylation are determined by lung ventilation, diffusion, and perfusion.

Total minute ventilation equals the total exhaled gas volume that leaves the lungs every minute. The volume of gas that reaches the alveoli and takes part in gas exchange is known as alveolar ventilation; the volume that does not take part in gas exchange is known as the dead space: the volume of the airways determines the anatomical dead space (about 100–150 ml for adults), and the number of non-perfused alveolar units determines the alveolar dead space [1].

Oxygen and CO_2 diffuse between the pulmonary capillaries and the alveoli. Diffusion is a process that depends on the partial pressures of gas on each compartment and a diffusion constant determined by the gas and tissue properties (e.g., CO_2 diffusion through the alveolocapillary membrane is 20 times faster than oxygen diffusion). Under normal circumstances, alveolar partial pressure of oxygen (P_AO_2) is equivalent to that of atmospheric air (159 mmHg). Partial pressure of oxygen in the pulmonary capillaries (P_aO_2) reaches 90–95 mmHg (slightly less than P_AO_2) due to venous admixture from the returning systemic circulation (Fig. 5.1). The difference between alveolar and arterial partial pressures of oxygen (PO_2) is known as alveolo-arterial gradient, and it is increased in disease states. At rest, the partial

Fig. 5.1 Representation of usual partial pressures of oxygen in capillary, arterial, and venous blood

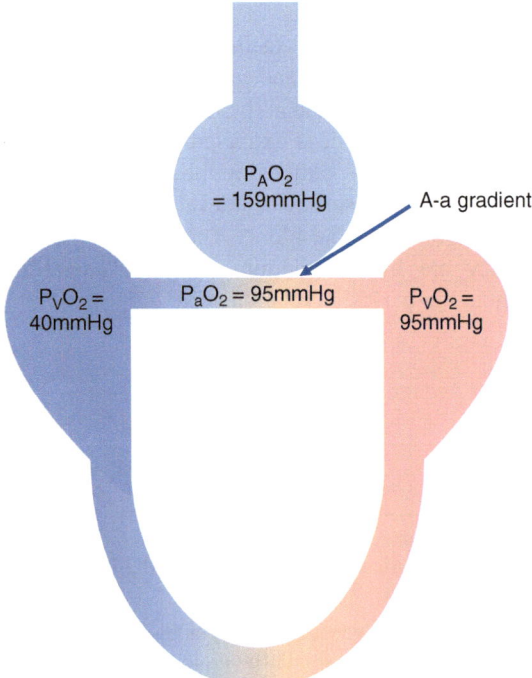

P_AO_2 = 159mmHg

A-a gradient

P_VO_2 = 40mmHg

P_aO_2 = 95mmHg

P_VO_2 = 95mmHg

Aerobic metabolism: O_2 consumption and CO_2 production

pressure of oxygen in blood reaches normal levels in approximately a third of the total time blood spends in the capillaries; during effort, capillary blood flow increases and the available time for oxygenation decreases. This can however be compensated by an increase in alveolar unit recruitment during effort [2].

Thus, the efficiency of the diffusion process depends not only on the difference of partial pressures, thickness, and surface area of the membrane (Fick's law) but also on the speed of the blood flow through the pulmonary capillaries.

Pulmonary circulation is a low-pressure system in which inlet pressure is the pressure in the pulmonary artery, outlet pressure is the pressure in the left atrium, and pulmonary flow is equivalent to systemic flow (in the absence of intracardiac shunts).

The passive determinants of pulmonary vascular resistance are blood flow, alveolar pressure, and lung volume. Increments in blood flow decrease pulmonary vascular resistance due to the recruitment and size increase of the pulmonary vessels. Lung collapse and high alveolar pressures increase pulmonary vascular resistance due to capillary collapse, which causes an increment in pulmonary artery pressures to sustain blood flow.

When alveolar PO_2 decreases, an active response mechanism called *hypoxic vasoconstriction* is activated. Small pulmonary arterioles constrict in response to alveolar hypoxia, and blood flow is redistributed away from poorly ventilated areas [3].

A balance between ventilation and perfusion in each alveolar unit is fundamental to maintain adequate gas exchange. The effects of extreme ventilation and perfusion abnormalities can be seen in Fig. 5.2.

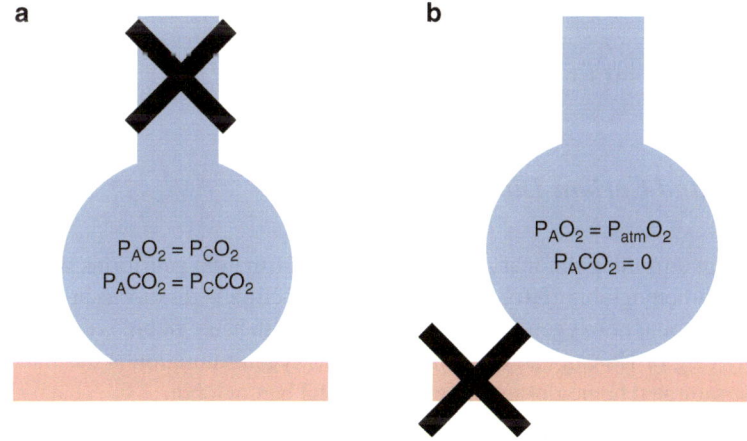

Fig. 5.2 (**a**) Represents a situation in which an alveolar unit is perfused but not ventilated, with a V/Q ratio = 0; (**b**) represents the opposite situation, a unit that is ventilated but not perfused, with a V/Q ratio = ∞. P_AO_2 alveolar partial pressure of oxygen, P_ACO_2 alveolar partial pressure of CO_2, $P_{atm}O_2$ atmospheric partial pressure of oxygen

In normal lungs, there are regional differences in gas exchange caused by the inhomogeneous distribution of ventilation and perfusion, with a ventilation-to-perfusion (V/Q) ratio which is higher in the pulmonary apex and lower in the bases due to the presence of a gravitational hydrostatic gradient, influenced by posture, lung volume, and application of positive airway pressures. In young and healthy individuals, blood is distributed to the areas with a V/Q ratio between 0.3 and 2.0 [1].

Patients with severe acute respiratory distress syndrome (ARDS) present with lung inflammation. The key histological finding is diffuse alveolar damage, which leads to alterations in the alveolocapillary barrier. This causes diffusion alterations, increased permeability with alveolar flooding, surfactant inactivation, microvascular thrombosis, and decreased lung compliance due to the closing of pulmonary units [4].

From a physiopathological point of view, ARDS causes both shunt and increased dead space, which lead to a lower partial pressure of oxygen in arterial blood (P_aO_2), depending on the amount of intrapulmonary shunt and the fraction of inspired oxygen (F_IO_2). Prone position modifies the distribution of aeration and perfusion, improves respiratory mechanics, and is associated with a survival benefit [5]. However, if intrapulmonary shunt is severe and refractory to prone positioning (pulmonary shunt/total pulmonary perfusion >0.4), increasing the fraction of inspired oxygen (F_IO_2) will provide little improvement in hypoxemia and ECMO may be the only viable solution [6].

Severe microvascular damage, compensating mechanisms such as hypoxic vasoconstriction, and change in intrathoracic pressures caused by mechanical ventilation can lead to increased pulmonary artery pressures and acute right-heart failure, which is associated with worse outcomes [7]. The use of inhaled pulmonary vasodilators such as nitric oxide can provide a transient improvement in hypoxemia and pulmonary artery pressures by vasodilating ventilated regions of the lung, but does not reduce mortality and may cause renal impairment [8].

Oxygen and Carbon Dioxide Transport

After uptake in the pulmonary capillaries, most of the oxygen forms a reversible union with hemoglobin (Hb), and only a small fraction is dissolved in blood. The maximal amount of oxygen that can be combined with hemoglobin is called oxygen capacity (1 g of Hb can carry 1.34 ml of O_2). Oxygen saturation is the fraction of oxygen-saturated hemoglobin relative to the total hemoglobin.

Oxygen uptake and release depend on the affinity of hemoglobin for oxygen. Affinity decreases (oxygen release increases) in low pH and high partial pressure of CO_2 (PCO_2) environments (such as the peripheral capillaries) and increases in the opposite situation (alveolar capillaries) [2]. The Haldane effect describes hemoglobin's ability to carry increased amounts of CO_2 in a deoxygenated state as opposed to an oxygenated state.

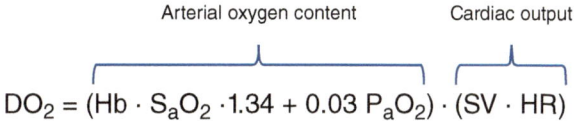

$$DO_2 = (Hb \cdot S_aO_2 \cdot 1.34 + 0.03\ P_aO_2) \cdot (SV \cdot HR)$$

Fig. 5.3 Determinants of oxygen delivery. For a 70 kg adult with a hemoglobin level of 12 g/dL, an arterial saturation of hemoglobin of 100%, a P_aO_2 of 80 mmHg, and an estimated cardiac output of 5 L/min, DO_2 would be approximately 800 ml/min. *Hb* hemoglobin, S_aO_2 arterial oxygen saturation, P_aO_2 arterial partial pressure of oxygen, *SV* stroke volume, *HR* heart rate

Carbon dioxide is a byproduct of aerobic metabolism. It is dissolved in blood (5–10%), transported as bicarbonate (60–90%), and bound to the residual amino groups of hemoglobin creating carbaminohemoglobin (5–30%). Due to the Haldane effect, the proportion of each group varies between arterial and venous blood [2].

The main determinants of oxygen delivery (DO_2) are the cardiac output (CO) and the arterial oxygen content. A detailed explanation can be seen in Fig. 5.3.

Under baseline conditions, the oxygen uptake ratio (VO_2) from capillary blood is around 25% of the total oxygen delivery (estimating a metabolic rate of 3–4 ml/kg/min for O_2). The respiratory exchange ratio is the ratio between the metabolic production of CO_2 and the uptake of O_2 and varies depending on the metabolism (usual range 0.8–1, although it can exceed 1 during intense exercise).

Experimental studies in humans and animals show that VO_2 becomes delivery dependent at DO_2 levels under 300 ml/min·m^2, a threshold called *physiologic supply dependency* [9]. Above this threshold, VO_2 is determined mainly by the cellular metabolic rate over variable DO_2 levels.

The metabolic rate is increased by sympathetic activation and stressors such as trauma, burns, surgery, sepsis, pain, agitation, and hyperthermia and decreased using sedatives, analgesics, and muscle relaxants.

A sustained disbalance between DO_2 and VO_2 causes tissue hypoxia and leads to organ damage.

Ventilation Control

Ventilation is regulated by the respiratory center in the medulla oblongata and the apneustic and pneumotaxic centers in the pons. A summary of their functions can be seen in Fig. 5.4.

The respiratory centers receive information from the central chemoreceptors located in the ventral surface of the medulla oblongata (sensitive to the changes in the concentration of H$^+$ in cerebrospinal fluid), the peripheral chemoreceptors in the carotid bifurcation (sensitive to changes in arterial PO_2 and PCO_2), and the mechanoreceptors in the lung. The role of lung stretch and baroreceptors is especially relevant, as they create a feedback mechanism in which insufflation and disinflation of the lungs inhibit and activate the inspiratory muscles.

Fig. 5.4 Respiratory control in the central nervous system

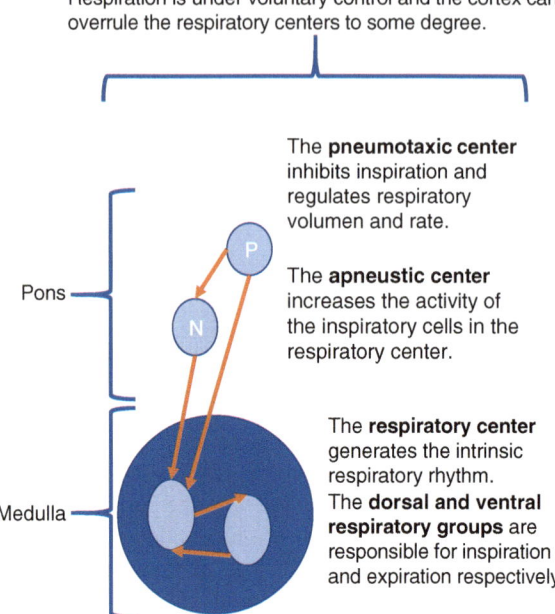

Respiration is under voluntary control and the cortex can overrule the respiratory centers to some degree.

Pons

The **pneumotaxic center** inhibits inspiration and regulates respiratory volumen and rate.

The **apneustic center** increases the activity of the inspiratory cells in the respiratory center.

Medulla

The **respiratory center** generates the intrinsic respiratory rhythm.
The **dorsal and ventral respiratory groups** are responsible for inspiration and expiration respectively

In ARDS patients, from a ventilation control point of view, both inflammation and increased work of breathing caused by low compliance and microatelectasis lead to a high respiratory drive. Excessive effort may cause patient self-inflicted lung injury even in non-mechanically ventilated patients [10].

Respiratory Mechanics

Movement of the respiratory muscles and the chest wall is required to achieve lung inflation. Two key concepts are compliance (a measure of the chest expandability, or the change in volume per unit of pressure, measured ml/cmH$_2$O) and elastance (a measure of the chest collapsibility, or 1/compliance).

Compliance changes during the respiratory cycle, being lower at volumes close to the residual volume and the total lung capacity: at low volumes, a higher pressure is required to overcome the collapse of the small airways and the surface tension of the liquid interface of the collapsed alveoli, whereas in hyperinflation, resistance to further inflation is greater.

In ARDS patients, lung compliance is determined by the amount of aerated lung units (functional lung size). High driving pressure (ratio between tidal volume and compliance of the respiratory system) stratifies mortality risk. Decreases in driving pressure owing to changes in ventilator settings or interventions are associated with increased survival [11]. Compliance can be improved by the recruitment of new pulmonary units or the improved mechanical characteristics of the already opened ones in the volume-pressure curve. Optimization can be achieved using higher levels of positive end-expiratory pressure (PEEP) and prone positioning [12]. However, in severe ARDS cases, maintaining a life-sustaining gas exchange may be incompatible with a protective ventilation strategy. These patients may benefit from ECMO support.

Work of breathing describes the energy required to ventilate and is associated with inspiratory effort, as expiration is usually passive. However, in cases in which expiration is active (such as air trapping), it can contribute significantly to the total energy expenditure. As work of breathing increases, so does the metabolic demand and oxygen cosumption of the respiratory muscles. In high work of breathing settings, respiratory muscles may eventually reach a threshold for fatigue, after which respiratory effort cannot be sustained for long periods of time [13].

ECMO Physiology

After VV-ECMO support initiation, oxygenation and decarboxylation depend on the ECMO flow and its interaction with cardiac output and residual lung function. Oxygenated blood is delivered to the right atrium and mixes with venous blood, increasing its oxygen and decreasing its carbon dioxide content. Total arterial PO_2 is equivalent to the mixed venous PO_2 plus the oxygenation delivered by the residual pulmonary function.

VV-ECMO has no direct hemodynamic effect as the volume of blood extracted and reinfused into the venous system is the same, so there are no modifications on central venous volume, pressure, or right ventricle preload. It does, however, produce indirect hemodynamic effects by decreasing right ventricular afterload (improving pulmonary vasoconstriction and allowing a reduction in ventilatory support and intrathoracic pressure) and reverting myocardial stunning caused by hypoxemia [14].

ECMO Oxygen Delivery and CO_2 Clearance

Membrane oxygenators perfuse venous blood through a network of small hollow fibers. The tubes are filled with flowing gas (oxygen or an air/oxygen mix), allowing gas diffusion across a membrane following Fick's law. Oxygen transfer capacity depends on the surface area and thickness of the membrane, transmembrane PO_2 gradient, and blood flow [15]. A graphic representation can be seen in Fig. 5.5.

The rated flow of an oxygenator is an estimate of the maximum oxygenation capacity under ideal conditions and is defined as the maximum standardized venous flow (Hb 12 g/dL, initial saturation 75%) that can be oxygenated to a saturation of 95% [16]. A comparison of the characteristics of different adult commercial oxygenators can be seen in Table 5.1.

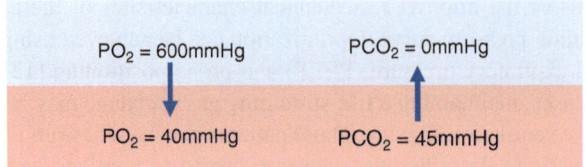

Fig. 5.5 Typical PO_2 and PCO_2 concentrations in the blood and air sides of a membrane lung (represented by red and blue color, respectively). Even though the O_2 gradient (600 to 0 mmHg) is much greater than the CO_2 gradient (45 to 0 mmHg), the solubility and diffusivity of CO_2 are greater, and the amount of O_2 and CO_2 exchanged is roughly equal at a gas flow-to-blood flow ratio of 1. If gas flow is increased to higher ratios, much more CO_2 can be removed. The gas flow-to-blood flow ratio is set according to the objective $PaCO_2$. Rapid decreases of $PaCO_2$ are associated with neurological complications due to alterations in cerebral blood flow, so hypercapnia should be corrected over 4–8 h after ECMO initiation

Table 5.1 Comparison of rated flows and surface areas of different oxygenators

Device	Getinge HLS 5.0 set advanced	Getinge HLS 7.0 set advanced	Xenios XLUNG kit 230	Xenios iLA membrane ventilator	Eurosets adult
Surface area	1.3 m²	1.8 m²	1.9 m²	1.3 m²	1.81m²
Rated flow	5 L/min	7 L/min	7 L/min	4.5 L/min	7 L/min

Table 5.2 Example of recirculation. Calculations are made assuming the following values: hemoglobin = 10 g/dL, pre-oxygenator saturation = 60% (baseline) and 90% (recirculation), pre-oxygenator PO_2 = 40 mmHg (baseline) and 60 mmHg (recirculation), post-oxygenator saturation = 100% (PO_2 = 500 mmHg) in both settings

Situation	Pre-oxygenator oxygen content (ml/dL)	Post-oxygenator oxygen content (ml/dL)	Oxygen added (ml/dL)
Baseline	8.3	15.2	6.9
Recirculation	12.4	15.2	2.8

If blood flow and membrane lung function remain constant, the main determinant oxygenation is the oxygen-carrying capacity of the blood passing through the device, which depends on the hemoglobin concentration and inlet blood saturation. An increase in inlet blood saturation (e.g., like in recirculation) decreases overall oxygen transfer efficiency and can lead to desaturation. A numeric example can be seen in Table 5.2.

Since blood is drained and reinfused in the venous system, a certain degree of recirculation is to be expected and should only be addressed when it is clinically relevant (e.g., compromised oxygen delivery). Baseline recirculation rates vary depending on the cannulation configuration, cannula size and positioning, direction, and speed of the ECMO flow and intracavitary pressures [17]. If necessary, it can be addressed by modifying any of the previous factors.

The most practical way of evaluating recirculation is to assess the trends of pre-oxygenator oxygen saturation ($S_{pre}O_2$) and arterial oxygen saturation (S_aO_2). An increase of $S_{pre}O_2$ with a fall in S_aO_2 may be an indicator for recirculation; $S_{pre}O_2$ can only be higher than S_aO_2 in the setting of recirculation.

Matching VO2, DO2, and ECMO

In a patient without any native lung function, systemic saturation will depend exclusively on the proportion of the ECMO flow compared to the total venous return (Fig. 5.6).

If cardiac output increases at a fixed ECMO flow, native flow will increase relative to ECMO flow causing a decrease in blood saturation. Oxygen delivery may increase due to the rise in cardiac output (Fig. 5.3). However, an increase in cardiac output usually happens in response to a hypermetabolic state, which may lead to higher oxygen consumption, generating an imbalance between oxygen consumption and delivery. This can be monitored for trending pre-oxygenator saturation (in the absence of changes in recirculation). Numeric examples can be seen in Table 5.3.

In general, after VV-ECMO, initiation flow should be titrated to the highest possible allowed by the current fluid status to assess maximal oxygen delivery capacity. The initial oxygenation goal is an arterial oxygen saturation of 88–90% [18], although lower saturation can be tolerated if there are no signs of delivery/consumption imbalance.

Typically, VV-ECMO patients require flows varying between 4 and 6 L/min when they are fully supported, but achieving flows over 5 L/min can be challenging. The main determinants of ECMO flow are drainage cannula size and pump preload

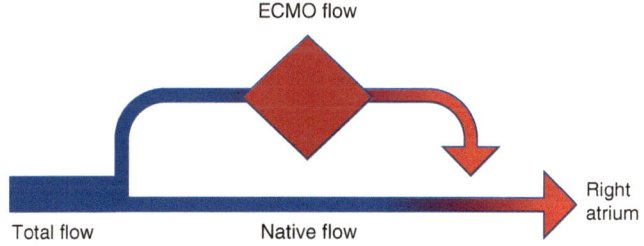

Cardiac output = venous return = ECMO flow + native Flow

$$Total\ oxygen\ content = \frac{ECMO\ flow\ O_2\ content \times ECMO\ flow + native\ Flow\ O_2\ content \times native\ Flow}{Venous\ return}$$

Fig. 5.6 Assuming no lung function, the total oxygen content will be the average of the oxygen content in the ECMO flow and the native flow relative to the venous return. This calculation can be done using saturation for simplicity, although it does not represent total oxygen supply, as it does not consider hemoglobin concentration

Table 5.3 Numeric examples of total oxygen delivery in different situations. Calculations are done assuming no recirculation, a total hemoglobin (Hb) concentration of 10 g/dL, ECMO $PO_2 = 500$ mmHg, ECMO saturation = 95%, venous saturation = 60%, venous $PO_2 = 40$ mmHg, unless otherwise specified. Physiologic supply dependency (threshold in which oxygen consumption becomes dependent on the supply) is around 300 ml/min

Situation	CO (L/min)	$Flow_{ECMO}$ (L/min)	$C_{ECMO}O_2$ (ml/dL)	$Flow_{native}$ (L/min)	$C_{native}O_2$ (mL/dL)	$C_{art}O_2$ (mL/dL)	DO_2 (ml/min)	S_aO_2 (%)
Baseline	5	4	14.5	1	8.3	13.3	665	99
Hyperadrenergia and pain	7	4	14.5	3	8.3	11.8	826	88
Anemia (Hb 7 g/dL)	5	4	10.6	1	5.8	9.6	480	100
Flow insufficiency	5	2	14.5	3	8.3	10.8	540	80

CO cardiac output, $C_{ECMO}O_2$ oxygen content in ECMO outlet blood, $C_{native}O_2$ oxygen content in native flow blood, $C_{art}O_2$ oxygen content in arterial blood, DO_2 oxygen delivery, S_aO_2 oxygen saturation in arterial blood (calculated)

(fluid status). Persistent positive fluid balance with the objective of maintaining high ECMO flows and increasing oxygen saturation should be avoided without signs of organ dysfunction, as ARDS management requires a conservative fluid balance [19–21], and the risks of a lower P_aO_2 [22] should be balanced against the known harms caused by positive fluid balance and increased blood trauma at higher blood flows [23].

Adding a second drainage cannula to achieve higher flows is an alternative in cases of small cannula size (stable but highly negative inlet pressure) but should be a temporary measure, as the differential flows across both drainage lines and turbulent flow caused by the Y-connector can lead to circuit thrombosis. The location of the extra cannula inserted is also relevant, as it may decrease effective flow by increasing recirculation.

When lung function starts recovering, arterial oxygen content and saturation increase, and the patient progressively tolerates lower blood and gas flows.

General Management of the VV-ECMO Patient

The care for VV-ECMO patients is complex and requires experienced teams [24, 25] and a flawless treatment of the underlying disease. VV-ECMO initiation provides organ support and promotes lung recovery by minimizing the aggressiveness of the mechanical ventilation and ventilator-induced lung injury. Patients with a severe respiratory impairment often require lengthy ICU and hospital admissions and suffer from long-term sequelae, so the goals of care during the ECMO run should be directed towards maximizing global recovery, with a strategy that promotes lung rest while encouraging safe, spontaneous breathing and rehabilitation.

ECMO-related complications should be actively monitored and treated, but the fear of complications should not lead to a premature removal of the ECMO support, as this may hinder global patient recovery.

Respiratory Management

Treatment of the underlying condition and avoidance of ventilation-induced lung injury are the cornerstones of the respiratory management in ECMO patients. Ultraprotective lung ventilation using low driving pressure, respiratory rate, and fraction of inspired oxygen (F_IO_2) should be established. Pressure control ventilation is the most common ventilation mode, targeting plateau pressures ≤ 24 cmH$_2$O, moderate to high PEEP (10–15 cmH$_2$O), respiratory rate of 4–10 breaths per minute, and $F_IO_2 < 0.5$. Passive patients in lung rest settings often present with impaired secretion clearance and may require bronchoscopy.

Prone positioning has proven benefits in the treatment of ARDS, but its role in VV-ECMO is still a topic of research. Retrospective studies show that it is safe and may improve oxygenation and respiratory mechanics, but also longer length of stay and ECMO duration [26].

After initial improvement, spontaneous breathing and active rehabilitation should be encouraged. At this stage, high respiratory drive and ventilator asynchrony should be carefully controlled to prevent self-inflicted lung injury. Transitioning ECMO patients from bed dependency to ambulation is feasible and safe when performed by trained teams [27].

ECMO Circuit and Patient Interaction

Blood exposure to the centrifugal pump, circuit, and oxygenator causes mechanical blood trauma, bleeding, and thrombosis.

Excessive mechanical stress (high rotation speed with inadequate pump preload, small cannula, and hypovolemia, or increased afterload and membrane thrombosis) is associated with hemolysis. Increased plasma-free hemoglobin levels cause organ damage by two mechanisms: direct renal tubular toxicity and nitric oxide depletion, which leads to increased vascular tone and abnormal platelet and coagulation activation. During ECMO support, severe hemolysis has been associated with mortality and an increased need for renal replacement therapy [28].

A certain degree of subclinical low-intensity hemolysis can be present without any relevant clinical manifestation. Acute and severe hemolysis may be detected by hemoglobinuria, manifested as a change in urine color (or effluent color for patients under renal replacement therapies). From an analytical point of view, plasma-free hemoglobin, lactate dehydrogenase, unconjugated bilirubin, and phosphate increase, and haptoglobin decreases. Trending those markers is recommended to detect potentially clinically relevant changes in hemolysis. If hemolysis is severe, a circuit change should be performed to prevent further organ damage.

Both hemorrhagic and thrombotic complications can coexist in the same patient and are associated with a significant morbidity and mortality [29]. Blood exposure to non-endothelial surfaces activates coagulation, fibrinolysis, and complement system. Venous thrombosis and clotting in the oxygenator and other turbulent areas of the circuit are common.

Clot formation can lead to decreased gas transfer efficiency (represented by a decreased post-oxygenator PO_2), impaired blood flow, and increased hemolysis.

Unfractionated heparin is the most widely used anticoagulant. A strategy to lower the risk of thrombosis and major bleeding usually involves highly protocolized anticoagulation monitoring using a multimodal approach [30]: various available coagulation tests (Table 5.4) provide information about different aspects of coagulation and often correlate poorly among each other.

Reports on the use of direct thrombin inhibitors such as bivalirudin and argatroban have been published in the setting of heparin-induced thrombocytopenia, but their use as the primary method of anticoagulation is not widespread [31].

Although continuous systemic anticoagulation is the current standard of care for ECMO patients, anticoagulation withdrawal is feasible and recommended in cases with high risk of major bleeding, such as polytraumatic patients; during the immediate postoperative period; or in case of severe thrombocytopenia. Moreover, there have been some observational reports on the feasibility and safety of routine anticoagulation-free ECMO runs with positive results [32, 33].

Table 5.4 Advantages and disadvantages of common coagulation tests and their usual goals in VV-ECMO (between brackets)

	Advantages	Disadvantages
aPTT (40–60 s)	Familiarity (historical gold standard for heparin monitoring) Widespread availability	Slow (30–60 min) Nonspecific (increased by low levels of coagulation factors, low fibrinogen, von Willebrand disease, and high CPR)
Anti-Xa (0.2–0.3 units/ml)	Specific (not influenced by coagulopathy, thrombopenia, or hemodilution) More efficient at achieving therapeutic range	Can be modified by hyperlipidemia and hyperbilirubinemia Has not proven improved outcomes compared to aPTT
ACT (160–200 s)	Point of care, commonly available Incorporates the effects of platelets to hemostasis Fast results (100–250 s)	Nonspecific (increased by thrombocytopenia, coagulation factor deficits, hemodilution) Inconsistency at low heparin doses
Viscoelastic tests	Point of care Fast (20 min) Provides information about fibrinolysis and heparin effect	Lack of sensitivity and specificity for heparin treatment adjustment

aPTT activated partial thromboplastin time, *Anti-Xa* anti-activated Xa factor, *ACT* activated clotting time

Table 5.5 Recommended tools for monitoring the patient-circuit interaction

Membrane lung status	
Post-oxygenator saturation	In the absence of clinical changes such as increased oxygen consumption (which leads to a lower inlet blood saturation), a decrease in post-oxygenator saturation can be a sign of loss of oxygenator efficiency. The two main causes are clotting on the blood side of the oxygenator or condensation in the air side of the oxygenator, which is more common when using low sweep gas flows and can be solved by increasing gas flow for a few seconds to remove condensation
Sweep gas requirements	In the absence of clinical changes such as deteriorating respiratory function, a progressive increase in sweep gas requirements can be a sign of loss of membrane lung efficiency
Pressure drop (Δp)	An increase in the pressure drop between pre- and post-oxygenator pressures (at similar blood flows) is a sign of increased blood flow resistance due to clotting
Visual inspection	The presence of clotting and fibrin in both oxygenator and circuit should be registered and monitored
Coagulation status	
aTTP, anti-Xa, ACT	Advantages and disadvantages of different coagulation tests are described in Table 5.4
D-dimer	A progressive increase in D-dimer can be a sign of higher thrombus load in the oxygenator
Fibrinogen	A progressive decrease in fibrinogen is a sign of incipient consumption coagulopathy. Refractorily low fibrinogen levels (<1.5 g/dL) should be a trigger for a circuit change in the absence of other causes
Signs of bleeding	New signs of diffuse bleeding (oropharyngeal bleeding, puncture-site bleeding) can be a sign of consumption coagulopathy
Hemolysis	
Plasma-free hemoglobin, total and direct bilirubin, LDH, haptoglobin	Routine diagnostic test for hemolysis should be performed. A degree of low-intensity hemolysis with uncertain clinical repercussion could be present. The goal should be early detection and prevention of severe hemolysis
Hemoglobinuria	Changes in urine color can be a sign of severe hemolysis

In short, daily clinical and analytical monitoring of the patient-circuit interaction should be performed. A summary of the recommended tests can be found in Table 5.5.

Summary

Severe disturbances in respiratory physiology can lead to life-threatening gas exchange impairment requiring ECMO support. After VV-ECMO initiation, oxygenation and decarboxylation depend on the ECMO flow, recirculation, and its interaction with cardiac output and residual lung function. Management of the underlying disease and ECMO-related complications is key for patient recovery.

References

1. Petersson J, Glenny RW. Gas exchange and ventilation–perfusion relationships in the lung. Eur Respir J. 2014;44(4):1023–41.
2. West JB. West respiratory physiology the essentials. 11th ed. Lippincott Williams & Wilkins; 2020.
3. Dunham-Snary KJ, Wu D, Sykes EA, Thakrar A, Parlow LRG, Mewburn JD, et al. Hypoxic pulmonary vasoconstriction from molecular mechanisms to medicine. Chest. 2017;151(1):181–92.
4. Bos LDJ, Ware LB. Acute respiratory distress syndrome: causes, pathophysiology, and phenotypes. Lancet. 2022;400(10358):1145–56.
5. Guérin C, Reignier J, Richard JC, Beuret P, Gacouin A, Boulain T. et al. PROSEVA Study Group. Prone positioning in severe acute respiratory distress syndrome. N Engl J Med. 2013;368(23):2159–68. https://doi.org/10.1056/NEJMoa1214103. Epub 2013 May 20. PMID: 23688302.
6. Sangalli F, Patroniti N, Pesenti A. ECMO – extracorporeal life support in adults [Internet]. Springer; 2014. Available from: https://link.springer.com/book/10.1007/978-88-470-5427-1
7. Zochios V, Parhar K, Tunnicliffe W, Roscoe A, Gao F. The right ventricle in ARDS. Chest. 2017;152(1):181–93.
8. Gebistorf F, Karam O, Wetterslev J, Afshari A. Inhaled nitric oxide for acute respiratory distress syndrome (ARDS) in children and adults. Cochrane Database Syst Rev. 2016;2018(6):CD002787.
9. Weg JG. Oxygen transport in adult respiratory distress syndrome and other acute circulatory problems. Crit Care Med. 1991;19(5):650–7.
10. Spinelli E, Mauri T, Beitler JR, Pesenti A, Brodie D. Respiratory drive in the acute respiratory distress syndrome: pathophysiology, monitoring, and therapeutic interventions. Intensive Care Med. 2020;46(4):606–18.
11. Amato MBP, Meade MO, Slutsky AS, Brochard L, Costa ELV, Schoenfeld DA, et al. Driving pressure and survival in the acute respiratory distress syndrome. New El J Med. 2015;372(8):747–55.
12. Guérin C, Albert RK, Beitler J, Gattinoni L, Jaber S, Marini JJ, et al. Prone position in ARDS patients: why, when, how and for whom. Intensive Care Med. 2020;46(12):2385–96.
13. Bellemare F, Grassino A. Effect of pressure and timing of contraction on human diaphragm fatigue. J Appl Physiol. 1982;53(5):1190–5.
14. Bartlett RH, Schmidt M, Brain M, Mauri T. The physiology of extracorporeal life support. In: MacLaren G, Brodie D, Lorusso R, Peek G, Thiagarajan R, Vercaemst L, editors. Extracorporeal life support: The ELSO red book. Ann Arbor, Michigan: Extracorporeal Life Support Organization. 6th ed; 2022. p. 73–95.
15. Bartlett RH. Comprehensive physiology. Compr Physiol. 2020;10(3):879–91.
16. Lequier L, Horton SB, McMullan DM, Bartlett RH. Extracorporeal membrane oxygenation circuitry. Pediatr Crit Care Med. 2013;14(5 suppl):S7–12.
17. Abrams D, Bacchetta M, Brodie D. Recirculation in venovenous extracorporeal membrane oxygenation. ASAIO J. 2015;61(2):115–21.
18. Brodie D, Bacchetta M. Extracorporeal membrane oxygenation for ARDS in adults. New Engl J Med. 2011;365(20):1905–14.
19. Seitz KP, Caldwell ES, Hough CL. Fluid management in ARDS: an evaluation of current practice and the association between early diuretic use and hospital mortality. J Intensive Care. 2020;8(1):78.
20. Ahuja S, de Grooth HJ, Paulus F, van der Ven FL, Neto AS, Schultz MJ, et al. Association between early cumulative fluid balance and successful liberation from invasive ventilation in COVID-19 ARDS patients—insights from the PRoVENT-COVID study: a national, multicenter, observational cohort analysis. Crit Care. 2022;26(1):157.

21. Wang YM, Zheng YJ, Chen Y, Huang YC, Chen WW, Ji R, et al. Effects of fluid balance on prognosis of acute respiratory distress syndrome patients secondary to sepsis. World J Emerg Med. 2020;11(4):216.
22. Barrot L, Asfar P, Mauny F, Winiszewski H, Montini F, Badie J, et al. Liberal or conservative oxygen therapy for acute respiratory distress syndrome. New Engl J Med. 2020;382(11):999–1008.
23. Kawahito S, Maeda T, Yoshikawa M, Takano T, Nonaka K, Linneweber J, et al. Blood trauma induced by clinically accepted oxygenators. ASAIO J. 2001;47(5):492–5.
24. Peek GJ, Mugford M, Tiruvoipati R, Wilson A, Allen E, Thalanany MM, et al. Efficacy and economic assessment of conventional ventilatory support versus extracorporeal membrane oxygenation for severe adult respiratory failure (CESAR): a multicentre randomised controlled trial. Lancet. 2009;374(9698):1351–63.
25. Riera J, Roncon-Albuquerque R, Fuset MP, Alcántara S, Blanco-Schweizer P, Riera J, et al. Increased mortality in patients with COVID-19 receiving extracorporeal respiratory support during the second wave of the pandemic. Intensive Care Med. 2021;47(12):1490–3.
26. Poon WH, Ramanathan K, Ling RR, Yang IX, Tan CS, Schmidt M, et al. Prone positioning during venovenous extracorporeal membrane oxygenation for acute respiratory distress syndrome: a systematic review and meta-analysis. Crit Care. 2021;25(1):292.
27. Cornman JB, Wells CL, Herr DL, Cypel M, Cucchi M, Schmidt M, et al. Physiotherapy and mobilisation. In: MacLaren G, Brodie D, Lorusso R, Peek G, Thiagarajan R, Vercaemst L, editors. Extracorporeal life support: the ELSO red book. Ann Arbor: Extracorporeal Life Support Organization; 2022. p. 607–21.
28. Dufour N, Radjou A, Thuong M. Hemolysis and plasma free hemoglobin during extracorporeal membrane oxygenation support. ASAIO J. 2019;Publish ahead of Print(NA):NA.
29. Murphy DA, Hockings LE, Andrews RK, Aubron C, Gardiner EE, Pellegrino VA, et al. Extracorporeal membrane oxygenation—hemostatic complications. Transfus Med Rev. 2015;29(2):90–101.
30. McMichael ABV, Ryerson LM, Ratano D, Fan E, Faraoni D, Annich GM. 2021 ELSO adult and pediatric anticoagulation guidelines. ASAIO J. 2022;68(3):303–10.
31. Kumar G, Maskey A. Anticoagulation in ECMO patients: an overview. Indian J Thorac Cardiovasc Surg. 2021;37(Suppl 2):241–7.
32. Kurihara C, Walter JM, Karim A, Thakkar S, Saine M, Odell DD, et al. Feasibility of venovenous extracorporeal membrane oxygenation without systemic anticoagulation. Ann Thorac Surg. 2020;110(4):1209 15.
33. Wood KL, Ayers B, Gosev I, Kumar N, Melvin AL, Barrus B, et al. Venoarterial-extracorporeal membrane oxygenation without routine systemic anticoagulation decreases adverse events. Ann Thorac Surg. 2020;109(5):1458–66.

Chapter 6
Physiology II: Venoarterial ECMO

Sagar B. Dave, Eric R. Leiendecker, and Christina Creel-Bulos

Introduction

Galen of Pergamon was the famed surgeon of gladiators. He was intimately familiar with those who rapidly approached death and detailed few of the first descriptions of cardiac and pulmonary physiology in those with critical shock states [1]. Since his work in the sands of the gladiatorial arena, the field of medicine has continued to pursue the understanding of cardiopulmonary physiology and manipulate it to save those who approach death. In this chapter, we will review our current understanding of cardiopulmonary physiology and discuss the role of venoarterial (VA) extracorporeal membrane oxygenation (ECMO) support.

Cardiac Physiology

A thorough understanding of normal cardiac physiology will help not only in the understanding of how patients get to the point of requiring mechanical circulatory support but also in understanding the complex interaction between the human body and the mechanical circulatory support system [2]. At the bedside, the cardiac

S. B. Dave (✉) · C. Creel-Bulos
Department of Emergency Medicine, Department of Anesthesiology, Division of Critical Care Medicine, Emory Critical Care Center, Emory School of Medicine, Atlanta, GA, USA
e-mail: sagar.bharat.dave@emory.edu; maria.christina.creel-bulos@emory.edu

E. R. Leiendecker
Department of Anesthesiology, Division of Critical Care Medicine, Division of Cardiac Anesthesiology, Emory Critical Care Center, Emory School of Medicine, Atlanta, GA, USA
e-mail: eric.richard.leiendecker@emory.edu

© The Author(s), under exclusive license to Springer Nature Switzerland AG 2024
A. R. Taha et al. (eds.), *ECMO: A Practical Guide to Management*,
https://doi.org/10.1007/978-3-031-59634-6_6

Fig. 6.1 Pulmonary artery
catheter showing the
location of injection port
and thermoister [3]

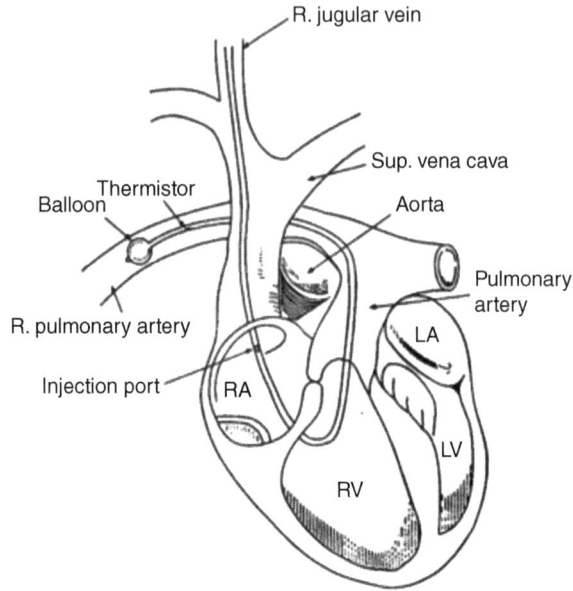

output can be measured either using a pulmonary artery catheter to perform thermo-dilution or drawing mixed venous oxygen saturations (Fig. 6.1). Thermodilution is a technique that uses a pulmonary artery catheter to measure the change in tempera-ture of fluid between themositers. Given the known temperature at the beginning and the measured temperature at the end, the only variable then is the time (or rate of travel) from one end to the other. Mixed venous oxygen saturation can be used utilizing the Fick's equation to calculate cardiac output [4].

One of the main determinants of cardiac output is stroke volume (SV)—volume ejected with each heartbeat. On bedside ultrasound, transthoracic or transesopha-geal echocardiography can calculate SV by obtaining two views—parasternal long axis where we measure the diameter of the left ventricular outflow tract (LVOT) and the apical five chamber where we can use pulsed-wave Doppler in the LVOT to obtain the LVOT volume time integral (VTI). If we picture the SV as a column of blood being ejected through the LVOT then, the LVOT diameter will yield the cross-sectional area of the column, and using the VTI, we know how far that column of blood moves in a unit of time. Thus, we can say $SV = (\pi r2) \times VTI$. By multiplying this by the heart rate, we have calculated the patient's cardiac output [5].

Variations in Cardiac Physiology

The heart rate can certainly vary to increase or decrease cardiac output though there must also be augmentation in stroke volume to effectively maintain adequate oxy-gen delivery to the tissues. This variation of stroke volume is the result of the

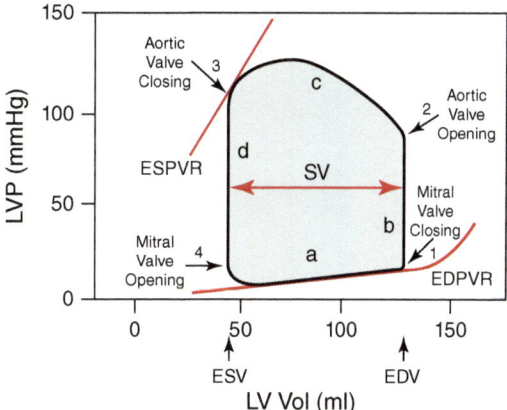

Fig. 6.2 Pressure-volume loop of the LV

balance and impact of three important factors: preload, afterload, and contractility. The best way to visualize the relationship of these variables, perhaps, is the pressure:volume loop (P:V loop) as seen in Fig. 6.2. Looking at the P:V loop of the normal heart, we can start at the bottom right of the curve (point 1), which denotes the end of diastole. Here, we see that the end diastolic pressure (LVEDP) is at the base of a vertical line [6]. This vertical line represents the isovolumetric contraction phase of systole, which terminates when the left ventricular systolic pressure exceeds the aortic pressure forcing the aortic valve to open and ejection to begin (point 2). Phase C represents the ejection phase where LV volume decreases as LV pressure increases to maximum prior to the LV starting to relax and the aortic valve closing again (point 3). From point 3, there is another vertical line, this time decreasing, indicating the isovolumetric phase of diastole. When this LV pressure falls below that of the left atrium, then the mitral valve opens and there is filling of the LV (phase A) where the LV volume increases and to a lesser extent so does the LV pressure [7, 8].

Within this graphical representation of the cardiac cycle, there are important physiologic principles on display. First, the stroke volume (SV) is displayed as the width of this loop—or the difference between the end diastolic and end systolic volumes. Second, the slope of phase A can also be described as the end diastolic pressure volume relationship, and this slope is the inverse of compliance. This means that changes in ventricular compliance can alter the slope of this curve such that increases in compliance flatten this curve and decreases in compliance steepen it. Third, the contractile state of the heart is defined by the end systolic pressure volume relationship (ESPVR). This is created experimentally by restricting caval flow and reducing preload, which leads to lower stroke volume resulting in a decrease in size and leftward shift of the PV loop. The ESPVR then is defined by the linear relationship of the points of end systole (point 3) of several loops with varying preload conditions. This definition dictates the maximal contractile force the lV is able to generate for any given preload.

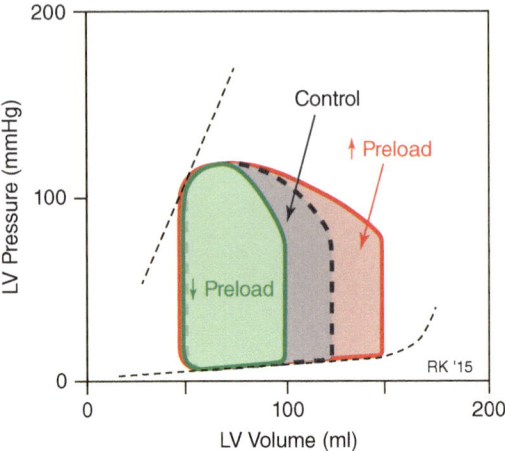

Fig. 6.3 Effects of preload on the pressure-volume loop

Turning attention to the question of preload, Fig. 6.3 shows how these PV loops can be used to show the effects of volume loading on the heart. Increasing preload will result in a higher left ventricular end diastolic volume (point 1). The Frank-Starling mechanism dictates the response in this situation, where the increased LVEDV leads to increased strength of contraction and larger SV. When LVEDV is increased, this is realized at the microscopic level by increased myocyte length, and thus sarcomeres are stretched immediately before contraction. This stretch translates in contraction to a larger contractile force to allow ejection of the increased volume. On the P:V loop, this is represented by a rightward shift of point 1 and the isovolumetric contraction phase, with LVESV being held static given no change in afterload or intrinsic contractile function. Due to a greater difference between LVEDV and LVESV, a greater stroke volume is produced and subsequently a higher cardiac output [9].

Conversely, the SV response to changes in afterload is inversely related where increases in afterload result in decreases in stroke volume provided that contractility and preload remain static. As aortic pressure increases, the isovolumetric phase of contraction prolongs due to the need for a higher LV chamber pressure to overcome the rise in aortic diastolic pressure. Because contractility is related to velocity of sarcomere contraction and due to the force-velocity relationship, there is a decrease in velocity of ejection. Assuming that heart rate, and thus time spent in contraction, is unchanged, there will be a lower volume of blood ejected in the same unit of time due to the lower velocity of ejection. Conversely, a decrease in afterload will allow for more rapid ejection and a larger volume of blood in a unit of time being ejected and thus a larger SV. Figure 6.4 shows how the P:V loop changes are represented by a narrowing of the loop (smaller difference between LVEDV and LVESV) with an increase in LV systolic pressures. With reduced afterload, this loop widens representing an increase in stroke volume with a reduction in LV pressures.

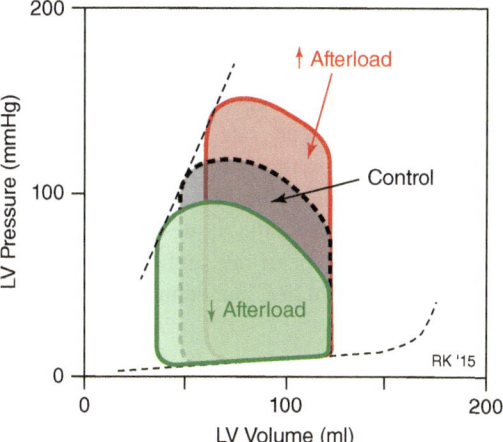

Fig. 6.4 Effects of afterload on the pressure-volume loop

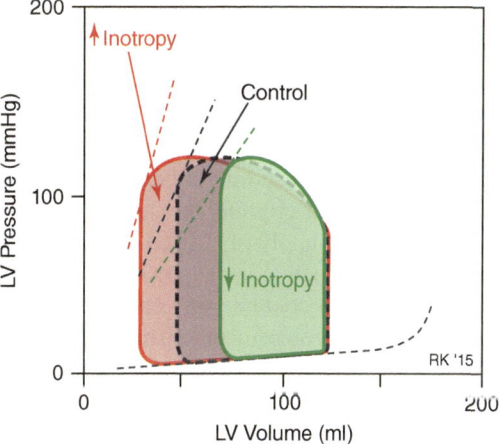

Fig. 6.5 Effects of inotropy on the pressure-volume loop

Contractility, or inotropy, can also augment SV by increasing the velocity of muscle fiber shortening. This leads to an increased rate of pressure and ejection velocity resulting in a decreased LVESV and an increase in stroke volume. Decreasing inotropy works in the opposite manner resulting in increased LVESV and a reduction in stroke volume. On the P:V loop, these changes are represented by changes in the slope of the end systolic pressure-volume relationship [10] (Fig. 6.5).

Changes in preload, afterload, and contractility can all alter stroke volume and the shape and position of the P:V loop. Changes in stroke volume will ultimately equate to changes in cardiac output and changes in oxygen delivery (DO_2), where increases in cardiac output lead to increased ability to deliver oxygen to the tissues and organs. If we consider for a moment the oxygen delivery equation, DO_2 = Cardiac output × Oxygen content. Expanding this, we see what variables are directly modifiable. Cardiac output can also be described as heart rate × stroke volume, where increases in either of these will lead to increases in cardiac output and thus oxygen delivery. We already learned that changes in preload, afterload, and contractility can increase stroke volume; now we see that if stroke volume is kept static, then changes in heart rate can increase or decrease the cardiac output as well. Oxygen content is the bulk of oxygen that is transported bound to hemoglobin. Increases in hemoglobin or saturation will increase the ability of blood to carry oxygen. Thus, DO_2 to the tissues and organs is directly proportional to cardiac output as dictated by heart rate and changes in stroke volume, hemoglobin concentration, and how saturated that hemoglobin is with oxygen [11].

Physiologic Goals of VA ECMO

The goal of this oxygen delivery is to meet or exceed the body's demand for oxygen. Oxygen consumption (VO_2) is derived from the difference between arterial and venous oxygen contents. This relation of supply and demand can be represented as the oxygen extraction ratio (O_2ER), which is the ratio of delivered-to-consumed oxygen ($O_2ER = VO_2/DO_2 = (SaO_2 - SvO_2)/SaO_2$). Under normal physiologic conditions, this ratio is low (~25%) and out of danger of creating an oxygen debt. As this O_2ER rises, consumption begins to rise and/or delivery falls, and the patient becomes at risk for crossing into anaerobic metabolism. A shock state occurs when there is an undersupply of oxygen delivery and an inability to meet the demands of the tissues. A reduction in oxygen supply may be due to either a reduction in cardiac output or oxygen content large enough to fail to meet the metabolic demand and resulting in anaerobic metabolism. This can occur due to a reduction in cardiac output from a multitude of reasons related to failure of the heart to supply enough stroke volume (changes in preload, afterload, or contractility) or a heart rate that is too slow. Shock state can also occur due to a lack of oxygen content in the setting of respiratory failure leading to lack of gas exchange, which would result in low arterial oxygen saturation. In these scenarios, the ratio of DO_2 to VO_2 is less than 2:1—there is a critical DO_2 threshold where the VO_2 is not being met and shock ensues [12].

Once these thresholds of O_2ER are crossed, there is a domino effect of cellular death leading to end-organ failure. Unless reversed, this end-organ failure will progress to multiorgan system failure and ultimately death. The purpose of VA ECMO is to provide restoration of DO_2 and lowering of the O_2ER back under that critical threshold. By optimizing cardiac output and improving oxygen content, O_2ER can be restored to an appropriate balance with the aim to stop the spiral of cellular death leading to multiorgan system failure and ultimately death.

Indications for VA ECMO

VA ECMO is a salvage tool that can be utilized in patients with critical, refractory shock [13]. It is important to recognize that ECMO in general is not a therapy but a supportive modality for salvage therapy in critical cases [14]. VA ECMO is no exception though it can support cardiac and pulmonary function. VA ECMO is performed with a cannula that is placed into a major venous vessel for drainage of blood that is pushed through temperature-controlled circuit via a pump, flowing through an oxygenator that allows for exchange of oxygen and carbon dioxide and returning through a cannula that is placed in an arterial vessel [13] (Fig. 6.6).

Though ECMO inherently aids in pulmonary function as the membrane oxygenation allows for gas exchange, VA ECMO specifically supplies support by providing perfusion to organs through arterial cannula return [16]. This can be helpful with disease processes that reduce cardiac output such as ischemic heart disease, stress cardiomyopathy, cardiotoxin overdose, accidental hypothermia, and arrhythmias—pathology that causes cardiogenic shock, where VA ECMO can be a valuable salvage therapy [17–20]. Similarly in pathology where cardiac output is reduced due to obstructive shock such as pulmonary embolism and traumatic pneumonectomy,

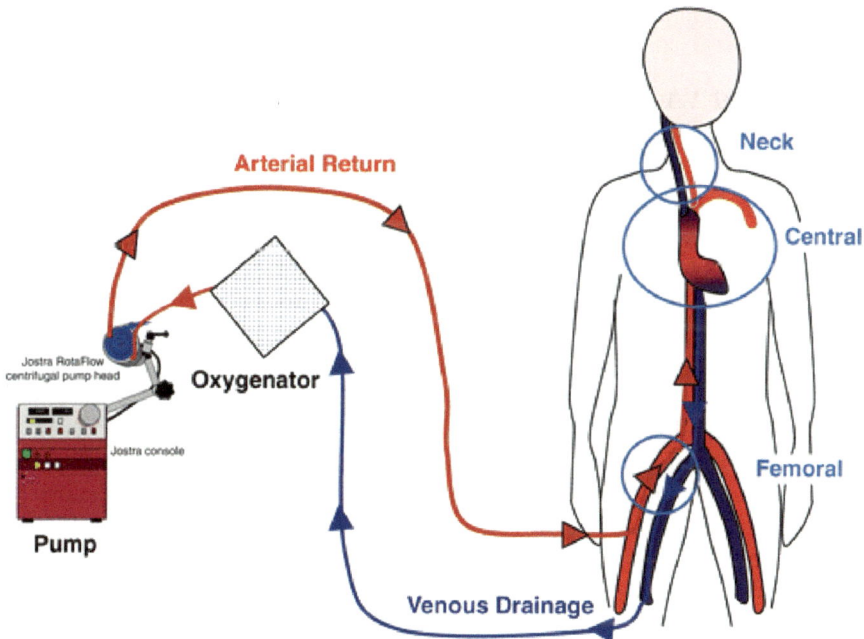

Fig. 6.6 Peripheral venoarterial extracorporeal membrane oxygenation [15]

VA ECMO can be helpful to reduce strain to the right ventricle and support perfusion in lieu of reduced cardiac output [21, 22]. Cardiac output can be potentiated due to right ventricular strain secondary to respiratory distress. In these scenarios, consider ECMO for respiratory support as the improvement in gas exchange alone can improve cardiac output [23].

VA ECMO is less successful in other areas of shock. Despite a surge of ECMO use in trauma, hemorrhage is still a contraindication of extracorporeal support [25]. Development of vasoplegic shock from spinal cord injury leading to neurogenic shock or infection leading to septic shock diminishes success with VA ECMO support as these pathologies are not primarily driven by reduced cardiac output [25, 26]. ECMO can potentially worsen these states with risks of infection, neurovascular injury, and coagulopathy [24, 26, 27]. It is important to consider favorable destinations of ECMO support. Favorable goals for the conclusion of ECMO therapy include recovery after intervention such as coronary stent placement or antitoxin. Other goals that require multidisciplinary coordination and time include heart transplant or durable left ventricular device placement. It is important to consider functional status, comorbidities, and variables that can contribute to overall prognosis [28]. The decision to proceed with cannulation in our program is always a multidisciplinary discussion. The burden of withholding ECMO, a potentially lifesaving support, should never fall on one's shoulders alone.

Initiation of VA ECMO

Initiation and cannulation for VA ECMO are primarily categorized into central and peripheral. Peripheral cannulation for VA ECMO can be performed at bedside or in a procedural suite [29]. Access can be done percutaneously preferably with dynamic ultrasound guidance or by cutdown for cannula placement [30]. In peripheral VA ECMO, the drainage cannula is placed through a proximal central vein for bicaval or transatrial drainage [29]. Certain systems also utilize a septostomy for biatrial drainage though this would require fluoroscopy [31]. The return cannula is placed ideally in the common femoral artery, which can lead to diminished perfusion and flow through the superficial femoral artery (SFA), which can lead to limb ischemia [32]. Limb ischemia in VA ECMO can be a large contributor for morbidity and mortality. Survival with limb ischemia decreases from 57% to 22%, and the risk of amputation ranges from 14 to 41% [33]. For this reason, a distal perfusion cannula is placed providing that antegrade flow is placed in the SFA and connected via Y-connector to the ECMO return tubing. Other options for distal perfusion include retrograde flow from the dorsalis pedis or anterior/posterior tibialis artery [32, 34]. For flow direction, a Hoffman clamp can be used to direct more blood flow into the distal perfusion catheter. Central cannulation involves sternotomy with drainage from the right atrium and return through the aorta. In central cannulation strategies, there is not a need for distal perfusion catheter as the cannulae are directly

connected to the heart [29]. Though this strategy mitigates the risk for limb ischemia due to cannula obstruction, it is much more invasive, can limit progression of
care such as extubation or physical therapy, and holds higher risk of infection and
bleeding.

Management of VA ECMO

Once cannulated for VA ECMO support, management is focused on providing systemic perfusion to prevent end-organ dysfunction while supporting diseased heart.
As mentioned previously, ECMO support aims to improve DO_2 to meet VO_2. With
flow of oxygenated and decarboxylated blood via return cannulae, coronary vessels,
cerebral vasculature, and other major organs are provided perfusion [35]. With this
consideration, it is important to maintain oxygenation through the membrane, optimize returned blood pH, and control temperature as this is the blood flow that is
required for end-organ function.

Identifying overall cardiac output and what is needed through VA ECMO can be
difficult to ascertain. Pulmonary artery catheter, which has been the mainstay for
measurement of cardiac filling pressures and function in various forms of shock,
can be skewed in VA ECMO. With falsely low pressures from blood diverted
through ECMO drainage, changes in temperature that confound thermodilution,
and effect on tricuspid regurgitation, pulmonary artery catheter measurements
should be scrutinized and accompany other monitoring devices to evaluate perfusion and cardiac function [36]. Cardiac output can be calculated and then added to
the ECMO blood flow for an overall cardiac output and oxygen delivery [37]. The
amount of cardiac output needed for perfusion is dependent on multiple factors
including patient size, metabolic demands, and various shock states. General goal of
ECMO flow is 60 cc/kg/min [38].

VA ECMO can also support a diseased heart by allowing for decompression of
ventricles that have poor contractility to minimize end diastolic pressure and progression of ventricular dilation. Flow can be increased to drain blood flow to the
ECMO circuit from native cardiac output, therefore reducing pressure in the right
ventricle, pulmonary vasculature, and left ventricle [39]. In peripheral VA ECMO,
this needs to be balanced with the risk of left ventricular overloading. As increased
flow through the ECMO circuit allows for drainage and diversion from native cardiac function, the afterload is increased and can lead to left ventricular distention,
elevated pulmonary capillary wedge pressure, and pulmonary edema or hemorrhage
[39, 40]. This balance of ventricle unloading and overloading requires vigilant and
continuous monitoring. Strategies for management of ideal ventricular loading may
include utilizing vasopressors, inotropes, or other mechanical circulatory support
such as temporary left ventricle assist device [41–43]. We will discuss these unloading or "venting" strategies further later in this chapter.

Anticoagulation on VA ECMO

Anticoagulation utilization in ECMO has become the standard of care based on the concern for potential extracorporeal associated hemostatic derangements and thrombus development [44]. Venous-arterial ECMO in particular places patients at higher risk for catastrophic complications related to thromboembolic phenomenon including but not limited to stroke, visceral infarctions, and associated organ dysfunction. In the setting of paucity or inadequacy of native flow, stasis and subsequent development of significant clot burden within the left ventricle, left ventricular outflow tract, pulmonary arteries, and pulmonary circulation can occur. Titration of anticoagulation to prevent hemorrhagic complications while preventing and managing thrombotic events can be a challenge [44].

As with all other indications for initiation of therapeutic anticoagulation, careful risk assessment and mitigation with respect to adverse side effects such as bleeding must occur. In the presence of clinically significant and/or persistent bleeding, modifications in the degree of anticoagulation can be employed [45]. In cases of life-threatening bleeding, ECLS support can be continued without therapeutic anticoagulation [46]. Ensuring that native pulsatility and ECLS flows through left ventricular and pulmonary circulation are balanced is paramount to minimizing thromboembolic risk [47].

Left Ventricular Venting

An increasingly recognized component of caring for patients on peripheral VA ECMO support is centered around the anticipation, early recognition, and assertive management of left ventricular (LV) distension. As mentioned previously, increasing peripheral VA ECMO flow can lead to supraphysiologic aortic afterload, which can lead to LV distension in the setting of reduced LV function. LV distension can subsequently result in a culmination of deleterious conditions including elevated left atrial and pulmonary artery pressures, development of pulmonary edema, pulmonary hemorrhage, and/or thrombus formation. Increasing LV wall stress and rising LV end diastolic pressure (LVEDP) can additionally lead to increased myocardial oxygen demands, resulting in subendocardial ischemia and further hindrance of LV recovery [47, 48]. Although risk of these complications is reduced in patients with a central VA cannulation strategy, this does not protect against the risk of root thrombus development and/or associated catastrophic embolization systemically or into the coronary arteries.

During instances in which a patient's heart is able to consistently eject blood through the aortic valve during the cardiac cycle, pulsatility is maintained, and pulmonary capillary wedge pressures remain low, additional LV venting may not be indicated. Medical management with utilization of inotropes/vasopressors, diuretics/renal replacement therapy, and careful titration of ECMO flows to the lowest acceptable level can facilitate LV decompression indirectly through promotion of the heart's native ejection of blood and reduction in ECMO flow-associated afterload. When these conditions are not met or when patients are struggling to meet an arterial pulsatility of greater than 10 mmHg between the systolic and diastolic values, LV venting should be utilized. Traditional methods for mechanical decompression of the LV range from percutaneous to surgically placed devices.

There are various options by which LV decompression may be accomplished. Considerations when selecting a device include not just the availability of the device and qualified operator to place the device, but also the underlying pathology compromising cardiac function, concomitant pathology, anticipated duration of recovery, and management goals (i.e., bridging and long-term options) of the patient.

Among percutaneous options, indirect (i.e., IABP) and direct venting (i.e., certain Impella subtypes such as the Impella CP) options exist. The IABP boasts a twofold benefit of augmentation of coronary blood flow during diastole in addition to decreasing afterload. Impella benefits include continuous drainage—from the LV with return into the ascending aorta—throughout the cardiac cycle independent of arrhythmias. Additionally, given its antegrade flow into the aortic root, it can prevent aortic root stasis, thrombus formation, and potentially devastating thromboembolic complications [49]. A myriad of other percutaneous therapy options can be performed with the aid of fluoroscopy. They include, but are not limited to, transseptal puncture with or without insertion of left atrial drain, transseptal septostomy, and percutaneous insertion of a pulmonary artery or retrograde trans-aortic catheter [50].

Surgically placed options include Impella 5.5—either placed independently or in conjunction with VA ECMO in "ECPella" configuration—and surgical vents that can be incorporated into ECMO circuit limbs [51]. The Impella (Abiomed, Danvers, MA, USA) is a miniaturized micro-axial flow pump driven by an electrical motor with an inflow cannula that directly decompresses the LV. Not only does decompression occur continuously through the cardiac cycle and independent of arrhythmias, but given its transvalvular location, it allows for continued coronary circulation [49]. Surgical vents can be additionally placed directly into the LV via the right superior pulmonary vein and then incorporated into the drainage components of ECMO circuit via a Y-connector. This is one of the most direct means of LV decompression; however, this must be meticulously placed [50].

Oxygenation and Hypoxia on VA ECMO

Until recently, no recommendations existed regarding the measurement of and parameters to define adequacy of oxygenation. ELSO guidelines specific to the management of VA ECMO now suggest avoidance of "excessive hypo- and hyperoxia" and monitoring right radial PaO_2 to detect the presence of differential hypoxemia [52]. Regarding the use of VA ECMO in resuscitation (ECPR), recent guidelines recommend "avoidance of hyperoxia" through blending of ECMO fresh gas flow with an air and oxygen mix," as well as "targeting a patient arterial oxygen saturation of 92–97%" [53]. The importance of monitoring for the presence of differential hypoxia in patients receiving VA ECMO support via peripheral cannulation strategy is paramount.

There are different etiologies for hypoxia in a patient on peripheral VA ECMO. Hypoxia can be noted in the setting of pulmonary edema from disease pathology necessitating ECMO therapy, but it can also occur in the setting of other conditions that can occur uniquely in this patient population: specifically, as a result of LV overload or differential hypoxia. Indications and methods for LV decompression in the setting of LV overload and associated pulmonary edema were previously discussed. Differential hypoxia, also known as "North South," "Dual Circulation," or "Harlequin syndrome," is a phenomenon unique to patients receiving VA ECMO via peripheral cannulation strategy. This phenomenon occurs as a result of retrograde peripheral VA ECMO flow competing with physiologic LV ejection of antegrade flow that occurs in the setting of myocardial recovery with concomitantly poor pulmonary function and gas exchange.

The result is the creation of an admixture of antegrade LV flow and retrograde ECMO flow, which leads to a transition point within the aorta. Depending on the location of this transition point in the aorta, reinfused well-oxygenated blood from the ECMO pump enters the distal portion of the aorta supporting abdominal viscera and lower extremities, while native circulation with poorly oxygenated blood perfuses the coronary arteries, cephalad component of the upper body, and can lead to cerebral ischemia, neurological complications, progressive left ventricular dysfunction, and ineffective ECMO support with significant hypoxemia.

Diagnosis of this syndrome can be made through obtaining directly invasive measures of oxygenation from the right upper extremity (i.e., arterial SpO_2 and/or PaO_2) and/or noninvasive methods (i.e., continuous SpO2 monitoring with probe placed on forehead). Basic management includes attempts to improve oxygenation via exogenous administration (i.e., mechanical ventilation) or temporarily increasing VA ECMO flow rates. The second can notably be counterproductive, as this increases afterload against which the recovering left ventricle must work. Other advanced options include conversion to VV ECMO if myocardial recovery is sufficient enough to liberate from VA ECMO and pulmonary function is sufficiently poor to require VV ECMO, or conversion to veno-arterial-venous extracorporeal membrane oxygenation (VAV ECMO) in the event that both cardiopulmonary support will be persistently needed for the foreseeable future.

RV Support

Right ventricular (RV) decompensation is a fatal complication that can occur secondary to many pathologies including, but not limited to, primary dysfunction or secondary injury such as left ventricular failure and/or chronic respiratory failure. The medical management of decompensated right-heart failure includes fluid balance optimization, inotropes, adjustment of mechanical ventilatory support settings, and usage of inhaled nitric oxide; however, in the absence of appropriate and/or sufficient response to medical management, mechanical support with ECMO or ECMO reconfiguration may be needed. There are many methods by which ECMO can provide RV support: options such as VA ECMO (VAV ECMO), right ventricular assist device (RVAD), and right ventricular assist device with oxygenator (Oxy-RVAD). The configuration used should depend on the presence and degree of cardiac and/or respiratory dysfunction [54].

Patients suffering from RV dysfunction can be at increased risk of device-related complications such as bleeding, thromboembolisms, and limb ischemia. These risks must be weighed against morbidity and mortality associated with the degree of RV failure present. Device selection and consideration should be based on patient-specific factors including duration of support needed, presence or absence of biventricular failure, valvulopathies, and tolerance of anticoagulation. RVAD and Oxy-RVAD have the ability to maintain physiologic anterograde and normal transpulmonary blood flow while additionally augmenting native gas exchange by way of membrane oxygenator in the latter [55]. As a result of cannula placement, both have been associated with significantly fewer systemic thromboembolic complications compared with VA ECMO and can be utilized without anticoagulation in cases of intolerance [46, 56].

Combinations in Extracorporeal Support

As the ECMO community continues to learn more about methods by which developing, expanding, and utilizing technology can be used to meet the complex needs of our patients, various combinations of extracorporeal therapy can be utilized with extracorporeal membrane oxygenation support. Commonly used combinations include ECMO and continuous renal replacement therapy (CRRT). Other options including combinations providing plasma exchange, leukopheresis, and molecular adsorbent recirculating system (MARS) have been cited [57].

Hybrid and Parallel ECMO Circuits

Hybrid ECMO circuits, or the expansion of the existing circuit to incorporate a combination approach (i.e., transitioning from venovenous ECMO to veno-arteriovenous ECMO), can be utilized when peripheral cannulation does not appear sufficient to meet patients' needs and augmentation of venous drainage or ECMO flow is necessary. Specifically, this can be utilized in the setting of refractory hypoxia or declining cardiac function to augment provision of support [58, 59].

Parallel ECMO circuit—the utilization of an additional drainage and return cannula connected to a separate VV ECMO circuit—is another method by which additional ECMO support can be provided. Examples in which this can be used include refractory respiratory failure in patients on VV ECMO with unusually high cardiac output states (i.e., sepsis) in which increased cardiac output may result in refractory hypoxia that is resistant to rescue maneuvers (i.e., beta-blockade, temperature control, paralysis, and proning). Similarly in patients on VA ECMO with flows insufficient for adequate end-organ perfusion or to promote waking and rehabilitation needed to facilitate potential bridging to transplantation, an additional VA ECMO circuit may be used to provide additional systemic flow and augment overall cardiac output to facilitate these goals [58, 59].

References

1. Lüth P. Galen von Pergamon [Galen of Pergamon]. Med Welt. 1965;36:2072–6.
2. Choi MS, Sung K, Cho YH. Clinical pearls of venoarterial extracorporeal membrane oxygenation for cardiogenic shock. Korean Circ J. 2019;49(8):657–77.
3. Tamura T. 5.05 - Blood Flow Measurement. In Brahme A. (ed.) Comprehensive Biomedical Physics. Elsevier, 2014;91–105, ISBN 9780444536334, https://doi.org/10.1016/B978-0-444-53632-7.00511-6. (https://www.sciencedirect.com/science/article/pii/B9780444536327005116).
4. Karpman VL. Die theoretische analyse der Fickschen Gleichung Zur Jahrhundertfeier der Anwendung des Fickschen Prinzips in der Physiologie [The theoretical analysis of Fick's equation. On the centennial of the use of Fick's principle in physiology]. Z Kardiol. 1975;64(9):801–8.
5. Nguyen LS, Squara P. Non-invasive monitoring of cardiac output in critical care medicine. Front Med. 2017;4(November):200.
6. CV physiology. n.d. https://www.cvphysiology.com/Cardiac%20Function/CF024. Accessed 5 Mar 2023.
7. Abraham D, Mao L. Cardiac pressure-volume loop analysis using conductance catheters in mice. J Vis Exp JoVE. 2015;103(September). https://doi.org/10.3791/52942.
8. Pollock JD, Makaryus AN. Physiology, cardiac cycle. In: StatPearls. Treasure Island: StatPearls Publishing; 2022.
9. Fukuta H, Little WC. The cardiac cycle and the physiologic basis of left ventricular contraction, ejection, relaxation, and filling. Heart Fail Clin. 2008;4(1):1–11.
10. Bastos MB, Burkhoff D, Maly J, et al. Invasive left ventricle pressure-volume analysis: overview and practical clinical implications. Eur Heart J. 2020;41(12):1286–97. https://doi.org/10.1093/eurheartj/ehz552.
11. Du Pont-Thibodeau G, Harrington K, Lacroix J. Anemia and red blood cell transfusion in critically ill cardiac patients. Ann Intensive Care. 2014;4:16. Published 2014 Jun 2. https://doi.org/10.1186/2110-5820-4-16.
12. Walsh TS, Garrioch M, Maciver C, et al. Red cell requirements for intensive care units adhering to evidence-based transfusion guidelines. Transfusion. 2004;44(10):1405–11. https://doi.org/10.1111/j.1537-2995.2004.04085.x.
13. Richardson ASC, Tonna JE, Nanjayya V, et al. Extracorporeal cardiopulmonary resuscitation in adults. Interim guideline consensus statement from the extracorporeal life support organization. ASAIO J. 2021;67(3):221–8. https://doi.org/10.1097/MAT.0000000000001344.
14. Dave SB, Deatrick KB, Galvagno SM Jr, et al. A descriptive evaluation of causes of death in venovenous extracorporeal membrane oxygenation. Perfusion. 2023;38(1):66–74. https://doi.org/10.1177/02676591211035938.

15. Butt W, Buckvold S. Extra-corporeal membrane oxygenation. In: Da Cruz E, Ivy D, Jaggers J. (eds) Pediatric and congenital cardiology, cardiac surgery and intensive care. Springer, London. 2014. https://doi.org/10.1007/978-1-4471-4619-3_178.
16. Lafç G, Budak AB, Yener AÜ, Cicek OF. Use of extracorporeal membrane oxygenation in adults. Heart Lung Circ. 2014;23(1):10–23. https://doi.org/10.1016/j.hlc.2013.08.009.
17. Abu-Laban RB, Migneault D, Grant MR, Dhingra V, Fung A, Cook RC, Sweet D. Extracorporeal membrane oxygenation after protracted ventricular fibrillation cardiac arrest: case report and discussion. Can J Emerg Med. 2015;17(2):210–6. https://doi.org/10.2310/8000.2014.141439.
18. Babatasi G, Massetti M, Verrier V, Lehoux P, Le Page O, Bruno P, et al. Severe intoxication with cardiotoxic drugs: value of emergency percutaneous cardiocirculatory assistance. Arch Mal Coeur Vaiss. 2001;94(12):1386–92.
19. Boue Y, Lavolaine J, Bouzat P, Matraxia S, Chavanon O, Payen JF. Neurologic recovery from profound accidental hypothermia after 5 hours of cardiopulmonary resuscitation. Crit Care Med. 2014;42(2):e167–70.
20. Chenoweth JA, Colby DK, Sutter ME, Radke JB, Ford JB, Nilas Young J, et al. Massive diltiazem and metoprolol overdose rescued with extracorporeal life support. Am J Emerg Med. 2017;35(10):1581.e3–5.
21. Pasrija C, Kronfli A, George P, et al. Utilization of veno-arterial extracorporeal membrane oxygenation for massive pulmonary embolism. Ann Thorac Surg. 2018;105(2):498–504. https://doi.org/10.1016/j.athoracsur.2017.08.033.
22. Conhaim JI, Levinsky NC, Barger PL, Palomino HL. Hybrid extracorporeal membrane oxygenation (ECMO) cannulation following traumatic pneumonectomy: a case report. Trauma. 2023;25(1):78–81. https://doi.org/10.1177/14604086211055288.
23. Grant C Jr, Richards JB, Frakes M, Cohen J, Wilcox SR. ECMO and right ventricular failure: review of the literature. J Intensive Care Med. 2021;36(3):352–60. https://doi.org/10.1177/0885066619900503.
24. Arlt M, Philipp A, Voelkel S, et al. Extracorporeal membrane oxygenation in severe trauma patients with bleeding shock. Resuscitation. 2010;81(7):804–9. https://doi.org/10.1016/j.resuscitation.2010.02.020.
25. Dave S, Cho JJ. Neurogenic shock. In: StatPearls. Treasure Island: StatPearls Publishing; 2022.
26. Falk L, Hultman J, Broman LM. Extracorporeal membrane oxygenation for septic shock. Crit Care Med. 2019;47(8):1097–105. https://doi.org/10.1097/CCM.0000000000003819.
27. Laimoud M, Ahmed W. Acute neurological complications in adult patients with cardiogenic shock on veno-arterial extracorporeal membrane oxygenation support. Egypt Heart J. 2020;72(1):26. Published 2020 May 24. https://doi.org/10.1186/s43044-020-00053-5.
28. Tonna JE, Abrams D, Brodie D, et al. Managements supported with venovenous extracorporeal membrane oxygenation (VV ECMO): guideline from the extracorporeal life support organization (ELSO). ASAIO J. 2021;67(6):601–10. https://doi.org/10.1097/MAT.0000000000001432.
29. Jayaraman AL, Cormican D, Shah P, Ramakrishna H. Cannulation strategies in adult venoarterial and veno-venous extracorporeal membrane oxygenation: techniques, limitations, and special considerations. Ann Card Anaesth. 2017;20(Supplement):S11–8. https://doi.org/10.4103/0971-9784.197791.
30. Cairo SB, Arbuthnot M, Boomer L, et al. Comparing percutaneous to open access for extracorporeal membrane oxygenation in pediatric respiratory failure. Pediatr Crit Care Med. 2018;19(10):981–91. https://doi.org/10.1097/PCC.0000000000001691.
31. Herlihy JP, Loyalka P, Jayaraman G, Kar B, Gregoric ID. Extracorporeal membrane oxygenation using the TandemHeart System's catheters. Tex Heart Inst J. 2009;36(4):337–41.
32. Ranney DN, Benrashid E, Meza JM, et al. Vascular complications and use of a distal perfusion cannula in femorally cannulated patients on extracorporeal membrane oxygenation. ASAIO J. 2018;64(3):328–33. https://doi.org/10.1097/MAT.0000000000000656.
33. Lamb KM, Hirose H. Vascular complications in extracoporeal membrane oxygenation. Crit Care Clin. 2017;33(4):813–24. https://doi.org/10.1016/j.ccc.2017.06.004.

34. Elmously A, Bobka T, Khin S, et al. Distal perfusion cannulation and limb complications in venoarterial extracorporeal membrane oxygenation. J Extra Corpor Technol. 2018;50(3):155–60.
35. Bartlett RH, Conrad SA. The physiology of extracorporeal life support. In: Brogan TV, Lequier L, Lorusso R, MacLaren G, Peek G, editors. Extracorporeal life support: the ELSO red book. 5th ed. Ann Arbor: Extracorporeal Life Support Organization; 2017. p. 31–47.
36. Su Y, Liu K, Zheng JL, et al. Hemodynamic monitoring in patients with venoarterial extracorporeal membrane oxygenation. Ann Transl Med. 2020;8(12):792. https://doi.org/10.21037/atm.2020.03.186.
37. Sistino JJ, Smyre JT, Patel K. Ventricular function determination during extracorporeal membrane oxygenation (ECMO) following Norwood operation: a case report. J Extra Corpor Technol. 2002;34(2):148–50.
38. Toomasian JM, Vercaemst L, Bottrell S, Horton SB. The circuit. In: Brogan TV, Lequier L, Lorusso R, MacLaren G, Peek G, editors. Extracorporeal life support: the ELSO red book. 5th ed. Ann Arbor: Extracorporeal Life Support Organization; 2017. p. 49–80.
39. Burkhoff D, Sayer G, Doshi D, Uriel N. Hemodynamics of mechanical circulatory support. J Am Coll Cardiol. 2015;66(23):2663–74. https://doi.org/10.1016/j.jacc.2015.10.017.
40. Choi MS, Sung K, Cho YH. Clinical pearls of venoarterial extracorporeal membrane oxygenation for cardiogenic shock. Korean Circ J. 2019;49(8):657–77. https://doi.org/10.4070/kcj.2019.0188.
41. Meani P, Lorusso R, Pappalardo F. ECPella: concept, physiology and clinical applications. J Cardiothorac Vasc Anesth. 2022;36(2):557–66. https://doi.org/10.1053/j.jvca.2021.01.056.
42. Shankar A, Gurumurthy G, Sridharan L, et al. A clinical update on vasoactive medication in the management of cardiogenic shock. Clin Med Insights Cardiol. 2022;16:11795468221075064. Published 2022 Feb 7. https://doi.org/10.1177/11795468221075064.
43. Cain MT, Smith NJ, Barash M, et al. Extracorporeal membrane oxygenation with right ventricular assist device for COVID-19 ARDS. J Surg Res. 2021;264:81–9. https://doi.org/10.1016/j.jss.2021.03.017.
44. Raffini L. Anticoagulation with VADs and ECMO: walking the tightrope. Hematology Am Soc Hematol Educ Program. 2017;2017(1):674–80.
45. Mazzeffi MA, Tanaka K, Roberts A, et al. Bleeding, thrombosis, and transfusion with two heparin anticoagulation protocols in venoarterial ECMO patients. J Cardiothorac Vasc Anesth. 2019;33(5):1216–20.
46. Olson SR, Murphree CR, Zonies D, et al. Thrombosis and Bleeding in Extracorporeal Membrane Oxygenation (ECMO) without anticoagulation: a systematic review. ASAIO J. 2021;67(3):290–6.
47. Ma C, Tolpin D, Anton J. Con: patients receiving Venoarterial extracorporeal membrane oxygenation should not always have a left ventricular vent placed [Internet]. J Cardiothorac Vasc Anesth. 2019;33(4):1163–1165. Available from: https://doi.org/10.1053/j.jvca.2018.11.007.
48. Werdan K, Gielen S, Ebelt H, Hochman JS. Mechanical circulatory support in cardiogenic shock. Eur Heart J. 2014;35(3):156–67.
49. Desai SR, Hwang NC. Strategies for left ventricular decompression during venoarterial extracorporeal membrane oxygenation—a narrative review [Internet]. J Cardiothorac Vasc Anesth. 2020;34(1):208–218. Available from: https://doi.org/10.1053/j.jvca.2019.08.024.
50. Cevasco M, Takayama H, Ando M, Garan AR, Naka Y, Takeda K. Left ventricular distension and venting strategies for patients on venoarterial extracorporeal membrane oxygenation. J Thorac Dis. 2019;11(4):1676–83.
51. Bitargil M, Pham S, Haddad O, Sareyyupoglu B. Single arterial access for Ecpella and jugular venous cannulation provides full mobility on a status 1 heart transplant recipient. ESC Heart Fail. 2022;9(3):2003–6.
52. Lorusso R, Shekar K, MacLaren G, et al. ELSO interim guidelines for venoarterial extracorporeal membrane oxygenation in adult cardiac patients. ASAIO J. 2021;67(8):827–44.

53. Richardson ASC, Tonna JE, Nanjayya V, et al. Extracorporeal cardiopulmonary resuscitation in adults. Interim guideline consensus statement from the extracorporeal life support organization. ASAIO J. 2021;67(3):221–8.
54. James L, Smith DE. Supporting the "forgotten" ventricle: the evolution of percutaneous RVADs. Front Cardiovasc Med. 2022;9:1008499.
55. Sertic F, Ali A. Acute-right-ventricular-failure post-cardiotomy: RVAD as a bridge to a successful recovery [internet]. J Surg Case Rep. 2018;2018(6). Available from: https://doi.org/10.1093/jscr/rjy140.
56. Oh DK, Shim TS, Jo K-W, et al. Right ventricular assist device with an oxygenator using extracorporeal membrane oxygenation as a bridge to lung transplantation in a patient with severe respiratory failure and right heart decompensation. Acute Crit Care. 2020;35(2):117–21.
57. Canter MO, Daniels J, Bridges BC. Adjunctive therapies during extracorporeal membrane oxygenation to enhance multiple organ support in critically ill children. Front Pediatr. 2018;6:78.
58. Shah A, Dave S, Goerlich CE, Kaczorowski DJ. Hybrid and parallel extracorporeal membrane oxygenation circuits. JTCVS Tech. 2021;8:77–85.
59. Pagani FD. Commentary: more is better: hybrid and parallel extracorporeal membrane oxygenation circuits. JTCVS Tech. 2021;8:86–7.

Chapter 7
ECMO Cannulation and Configuration

Ihab Ahmed

Introduction

A vital requirement for successful extracorporeal support is uninterrupted access to the circulation to maintain adequate blood flow and gas exchange. An inadequate extracorporeal flow can limit ECLS's potential benefits by not providing adequate support. Cannulation configuration, cannula size, and types of ECMO cannula are all influenced by the mode of support, patient size, anatomical features of the vascular tree, as well as institutional considerations. The purpose of this chapter is to provide an overview of both basic and complex cannulation techniques for ECLS.

Extracorporeal Support Cannulas

Various vascular access cannulas are available on the market. There are different types of cannulas, depending on the method of insertion (percutaneous or surgical), direction of the blood flow (drainage or reinfusion), as well as lengths and diameters to accommodate which vessel is being used.

Peripheral Versus Surgical Cannula Types

Percutaneous peripheral cannulas differ from those meant for surgical placement in some ways. Surgical cannulas have blunt dilators with short tips and no central lumen, while percutaneous dilators have a long taper and central lumen to

I. Ahmed (✉)
Critical Care Institute Cleveland Clinic Abu Dhabi, Abu Dhabi, United Arab Emirates

© The Author(s), under exclusive license to Springer Nature
Switzerland AG 2024
A. R. Taha et al. (eds.), *ECMO: A Practical Guide to Management*,
https://doi.org/10.1007/978-3-031-59634-6_7

accommodate a guidewire. Percutaneous cannulas are designed with a point that fits snugly against the dilator and is tapered for ease of insertion, unlike surgical cannulas, which have this feature as an option.

An embedded layer of spiral-wound metal wire reinforces the wall of the percutaneous cannula. As a result of this reinforcement, the cannula can flex without kinking, resist flattening under external compression, and risk collapsing under negative pressure. As a result, reinforced cannulas are generally preferred since complications can result in the loss of extracorporeal support.

Single-Lumen Cannula

It is further defined by the stages or holes available in the cannula, whether it is used for drainage or reinfusion.

A *drainage or access* cannula, which is commercially referred to also as a venous cannula, drains blood from the venous circulation into the ECMO circuit and usually has a greater length of up to 55 cm with multiple holes, which is referred to as a *multistage* cannula to facilitate venous drainage with less negative pressure. Different sizes of cannulas are available on the market (Fig. 7.1).

A *reinfusion or return* cannula, which is commercially referred to also as an arterial cannula, returns the blood back to the patient into either arterial or venous circulation

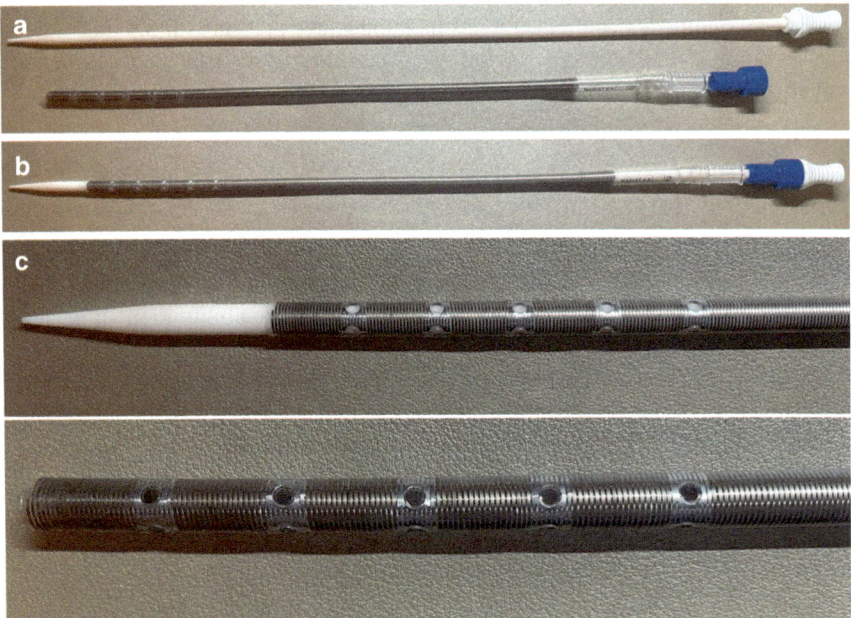

Fig. 7.1 Access or drainage cannula (commercially venous cannula). Picture (**a**) Drainage cannula multistage and introducer outside. Picture (**b**) Drainage cannula multistage and introducer inside. Picture (**c**) Multistage holes

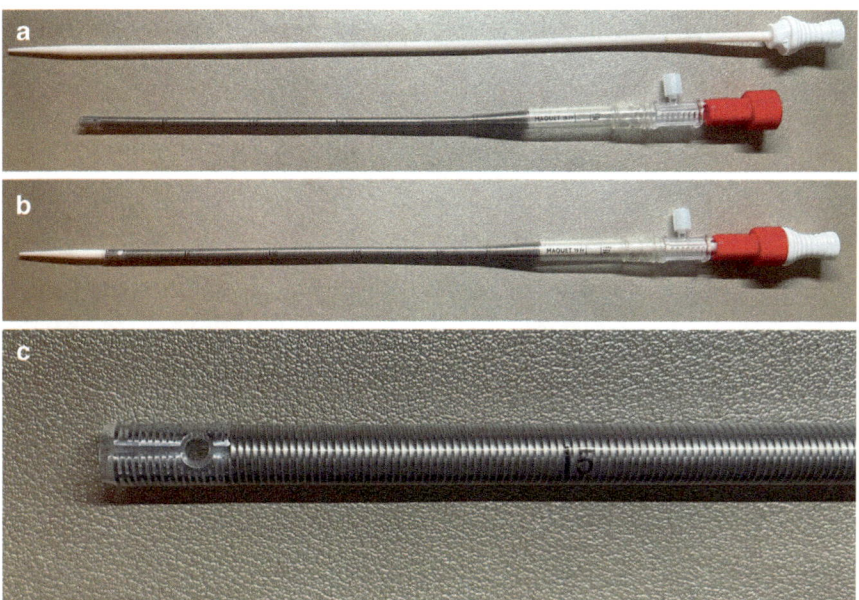

Fig. 7.2 Return or reinfusion cannula (commercially arterial cannula). Picture (**a**) Return cannula single stage and introducer outside. Picture (**b**) Return cannula single stage and introducer inside. Picture (**c**) Single-stage hole

according to the configuration and mode of support and usually has a lesser length of between 15 and 23 cm with a lesser hole, which is referred to as a *single-stage* cannula to allow laminar flow without turbulence to the designated destination. Different sizes and lengths of cannulas are available on the market (Fig. 7.2).

In some configurations, longer single-stage cannulas of up to 50 cm are required for reinfusion. See sections Fem-Femoral VV ECMO and Veno-Pulmonary Arterial Cannulation (VPa).

Double-Lumen Cannula

A line of dual-lumen cannulas designed specifically for placement inside the right internal jugular vein is currently being used in clinical practice. Among the commercially available cannulas are Avalon Elite® (Avalon Laboratories) and Crescent™* Jugular Dual Lumen Catheter.

The cannula is divided into two lumens by an inner membrane. A return lumen is positioned 10 cm from the tip of the cannula and is designed to return blood to the RA. There is a drainage lumen, with end holes and side holes at the tip located in the IVC, as well as side holes proximal to the exit site of the return lumen positioned in the SVC. Thus, it allows drainage from both the SVC and the IVC. Different sizes of cannulas are available on the market. See Table 7.3.

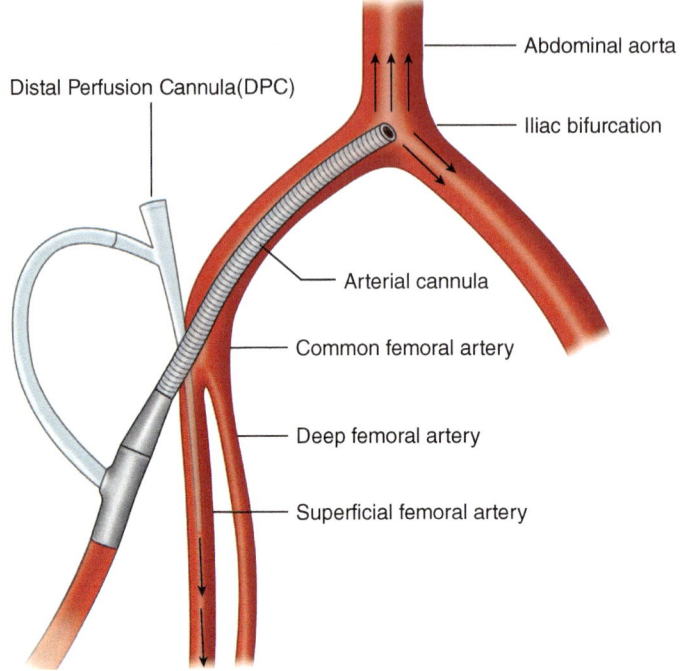

Fig. 7.3 Antegrade distal perfusion cannula

Distal Perfusion Cannula (DPC)

In essence, it is a reinforced catheter with a diameter of 5–8 Fr. It is inserted into the ipsilateral artery where the arterial ECMO cannula is inserted. An antegrade DPC is inserted into the femoral or superficial femoral arteries distal to the site of ECMO cannulation, whereas a retrograde DPC is placed into the dorsalis pedis or the posterior tibial arteries (Fig. 7.3).

How to Choose Your Cannula

ECMO cannula flow follows the same basic principles as any fluid flow in a tube and follows the Bernoulli equation, the simplified Poiseuille equation,

$$Q = \frac{\Delta P r^4}{8 \mu L}$$

(where Q is the flow rate, μ is the viscosity, r is the radius, L is the length of the cannula, and ΔP is the pressure across the cannula), which states that the maximum flow is inversely proportional to the cannula length and directly proportional to the fourth power of the radius for a circular cross-section cannula.

As a general rule, shorter and larger diameter cannulas are the preferred choice with respect to all the available factors.

Five factors affecting your decision to choose the cannula:

1. Size of the patient
2. Configuration that you will apply
3. Anatomical barrier
4. ECMO flow required
5. Vessel diameter

The *cannula length* is primarily determined by the patient's size and the ECMO configuration as cannulation near the heart usually requires shorter cannulas than peripherally inserted in the lower limb to reach the right atrium.

Cannula diameter is determined primarily by the vessel size and ECMO flow requirements, and flow guidance can be obtained from the manufacturer's chart. See Tables 7.1, 7.2, and 7.3 and their references. Prior to cannulation, 2D ultrasound

Table 7.1 Arterial cannula for peripheral ECMO

Manufacturer	Size in Fr	Length in cm	Pressure gradient at flow 3 L/min for 19–20 Fr	Pressure gradient at flow 5 L/min for 19–20 Fr
Getinge 1	13, 15, 17, 19, 21, 23	15	30	100
	15, 17, 19, 21, 23	23	45	120
Medtronic 2	15, 17, 19, 21, 23, 25	18	35	80
Edwards 3	16, 18, 20, 22	15	45	80

1-Getinge: HLS Cannulae Set·Instructions for Use 70104.8192 G-139 Version 05 NONUS 2021–04
www.getinge.com/dam/hospital/documents/english/hls_cannulae_brochure-en-non_us_japan.pdf
2-Medtronic: https://europe.medtronic.com/xd-en/healthcare-professionals/products/cardiovascu-lar/extracorporeal-life-support/bio-medicus-nextgen.html
3-Edwards Lifesciences: https://www.edwards.com/gb/devices/Catheters/Arterial-Cannulae

Table 7.2 Venous cannula for peripheral ECMO

Manufacturer	Size in Fr	Length in cm	Pressure gradient at flow 3 L/min for 25 Fr	Pressure gradient at flow 5 L/min for 25 Fr
Getinge 1	19, 21, 23, 25	38	15	35
	21, 23, 25, 29	55	20	40
Medtronic 2	15, 17	50	18	38
	19, 21	55		
	23, 25, 27, 29	60		

1-Getinge: HLS Cannula Set·Instructions for Use 70104.8192 G-139 Version 05 NONUS 2021–04
www.getinge.com/dam/hospital/documents/english/hls_cannulae_brochure-en-non_us_japan.pdf
2-Medtronic: https://europe.medtronic.com/xd-en/healthcare-professionals/products/cardiovascu-lar/extracorporeal-life-support/bio-medicus-nextgen.html

Table 7.3 Bicaval dual-lumen cannula

Manufacturer	Size in Fr	Length in cm	Pressure gradient at flow 3 L/min for 31–32 Fr	Pressure gradient at flow 5 L/min for 31–32 Fr
Getinge 1 Avalon Elite	13, 16, 19	11, 14, 21	–	–
	20–31	31	20 on drainage lumen 60 on reinfusion lumen	50 on drainage lumen 160 on reinfusion lumen
Medtronic 2 Crescent™	24, 26	30	20 on drainage lumen 50 on reinfusion lumen	40 on drainage lumen 120 on reinfusion lumen
	28, 30, 32	34		

1-Getinge: www.getinge.com/dam/hospital/documents/english/avalon_elite_brochure-en-non_us.pdf
2-Medtronic: https://europe.medtronic.com/xd-en/healthcare-professionals/products/cardiovascu-lar/extracorporeal-life-support/crescent-jugular-dual-lumen-catheter.html

imaging is performed to assess vessel size and patency at potential sites of cannulation. Compressibility and Doppler color flow are used to verify vein patency. Vein diameters are then measured, with vein size calculated from the formula:

$$Size(Fr) = D(mm) \times 3$$

If the vein contour is distorted from adjacent tissue, the size (Fr) is calculated as the circumference of the vein in millimeters. For femoral arterial cannulation, the arterial lumen diameter is determined as for the vein. Cannulas chosen for insertion are selected to be at least 1–3F sizes smaller than the calculated vessel size for pediatric or adult patients, respectively [7].

ECMO Cannula Configurations

Cannulation configuration is primarily determined by the mode of support and vascular access. A venoarterial ECMO (VA ECMO) configuration was historically used to provide extracorporeal life support for both respiratory and cardiac failure. While still the preferred configuration for cardiac failure, the venovenous ECMO (VV ECMO) configuration, along with other configurations, has been developed that is more suitable for other types of support.

Conventional Configurations

VV ECMO Configurations

The venous blood is drained from the central veins and then circulated through the oxygenator so that oxygenated blood can enter the venous system, and it uses the native cardiac function for oxygen delivery to the whole body. The goal of VV

ECMO cannula configurations is to maximize flow and minimize recirculation. The preferred way to achieve high flow rates is to place a large drainage cannula, and in order to minimize recirculation, oxygenated blood should be returned to the RA, ideally with the flow directed through the tricuspid valve. Following is an overview of the configurations used.

Fem-Jugular VV ECMO

A multistage drainage cannula is inserted into the femoral vein and advanced through the IVC, and a single-stage return cannula is inserted into the jugular vein with the tip ends by the SVC-right atrium junction. The right side is preferred as it provides a straight path inside these vessels, although either side can be used. Ideally, the access cannula tip should be positioned in the hepatic portion of the IVC between the hepatic vein junction and the IVC-right atrium junction. The tips of the drainage and return cannulas should be separated by at least 10 cm to minimize recirculation. This is a condition where the infused oxygenated blood is recirculated into the drainage cannula without entering the heart. A return cannula length of 15 cm is the optimum choice to be placed at the SVC-RT atrial junction in order to prevent cannula redundancy in the right atrium causing arrhythmias or injuries. In cases where the left IJ vein will be cannulated, a taller cannula can be utilized as long as the patient is not too small (Fig. 7.4).

Fem-Femoral VV ECMO

Both femoral veins will be cannulated in this configuration. One of the femoral veins is used for the insertion of a multistage drainage cannula, which will be located below the diaphragm and above the renal veins, while the other femoral vein is used for the insertion of a longer single-stage return cannula to reach the right atrium, typically 50–60 cm long. In the IVC, both cannulas share the same space. As mentioned above, the tips of the two cannulas should be separated by at least 10 cm in order to minimize recirculation.

A disadvantage of this configuration is that both cannulas are in the groin. This limits the patient to sitting in bed, increasing the risk of infection and carrying the highest rate of recirculation. This is given that both cannulas are in IVC. Another issue with this configuration is that the drainage cannula level must be low in IVC compared to the fem-jugular approach, usually between hepatic and renal vein opening in IVC, which makes this cannula vulnerable to changes to intra-abdominal pressure that may preclude venous drainage. As mentioned earlier, given that both cannulas share the same space in IVC, this may limit the size of cannulas used (Fig. 7.5).

Fig. 7.4 Fem-jugular
approach in VV ECMO
configuration

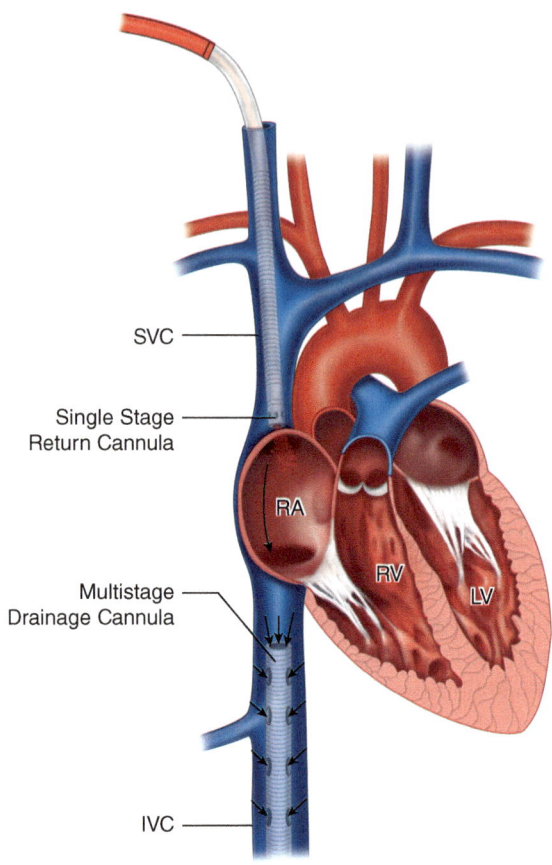

Bicaval Dual-Lumen Cannulation

The bicaval dual-lumen cannula is designed where only one vein needs to be cannulated: the right internal jugular vein [1]. However, there are reports of using the left subclavian veins in patients where the right IJ vein cannot be used [10, 11].

As previously mentioned in the section describing cannula types, this cannula has two lumens, one for drainage and one for return. The drainage hole is located in the SVC and IVC. The return hole is located in the right atrium and faces the tricuspid valve. It is imperative that the cannula is positioned appropriately by transesophageal echocardiography so that the jet of blood that emerges from the return hole is directed toward the tricuspid valve.

An advantage of the bicaval dual-lumen cannula is that one-site cannulation can be easily managed during rehabilitation and physiotherapy in patients who are required to be on ECMO for an extended period. As a result, most of the time, it is the configuration of choice for patients undergoing lung transplants, and awake

Fig. 7.5 Fem-femoral
approach in VV ECMO
configuration

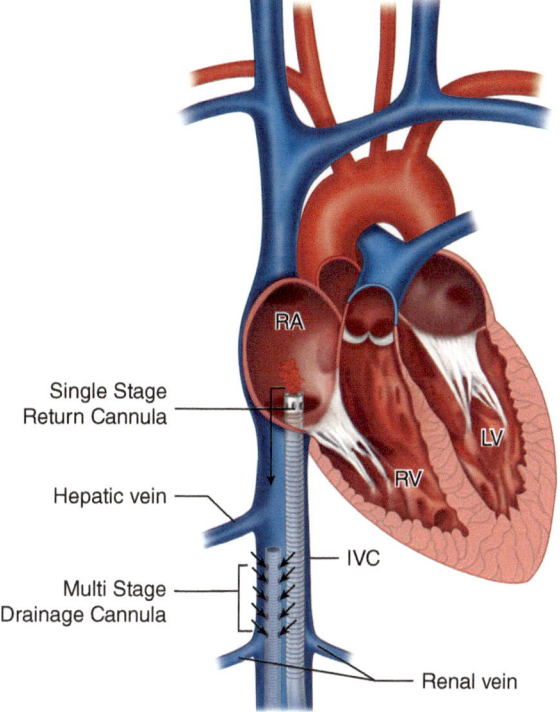

insertion can be performed. Unlike femoral site cannulation, this allows the patient to sit and walk freely, with less infection than groin-site cannulation. In addition, it is the least configuration with recirculation if the cannula is positioned correctly.

It should be pointed out that one of the major *disadvantages* associated with the bicaval dual-lumen cannula is its limitation of flow, even with the largest diameter. This is particularly true when the patient is large or high ECMO flows exceeding 5 liters are required. In this case, double-site cannulation would be more appropriate. Furthermore, any movement of the cannula may allow it to be displaced proximally or distally, which will allow it to change the position of the return hole, which may result in significant recirculation and/or low blood flow, which may result in hypoxia (Fig. 7.6).

Veno-Pulmonary Arterial Cannulation (VPa)

In order to fulfill this section, this is just a description of a very recent modification of VV ECMO that has not been validated in studies. The purpose of VPa ECMO is the same as that of VV ECMO cannulation: to drain the venous blood from the right atrium and supply the reoxygenated and decarboxylated blood back into the pulmonary circulation. Unlike VV ECMO, the return cannula does not terminate in the

Fig. 7.6 Bicaval
dual-lumen cannula
approach in VV ECMO
configuration

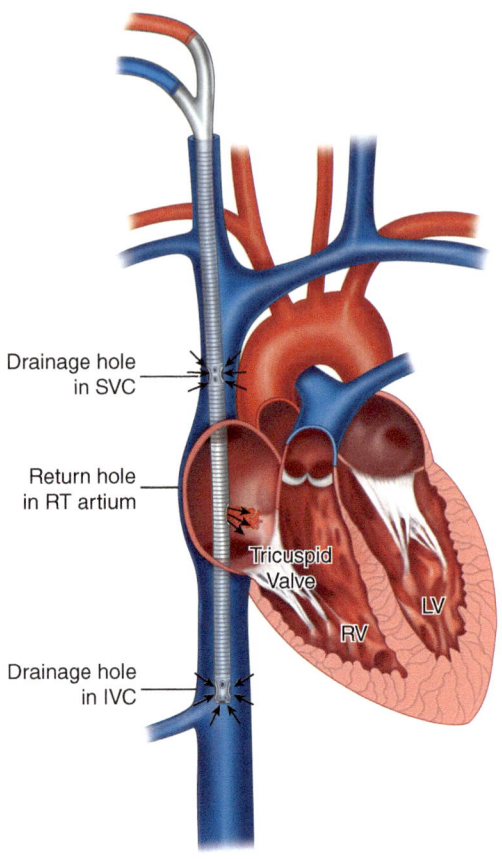

Fig. 7.6 Bicaval dual-lumen cannula approach in VV ECMO configuration

right atrium but rather travels through the tricuspid valve, the right ventricle, and the pulmonary valve to reach the pulmonary artery. Consequently, this cannulation bypasses the right ventricle, which in turn is used to treat patients with isolated right-heart failure or right-heart failure that occurred during VV ECMO treatment (Fig. 7.7).

VA ECMO Configurations

VA ECMO is typically a high-flow heart-lung machine providing calculated full flow up to 2.5 L/m2/min. Usually, venous blood is drained from the right atrium. The blood is pumped through a membrane oxygenator allowing oxygen to be added and carbon dioxide to be removed and returned to the systemic arterial circulation. This VA ECMO configuration is a closed circuit that bypasses the lungs and heart, supporting severe cardiac failure with or without concomitant respiratory failure. There are two principal VA ECMO configurations, central and peripheral.

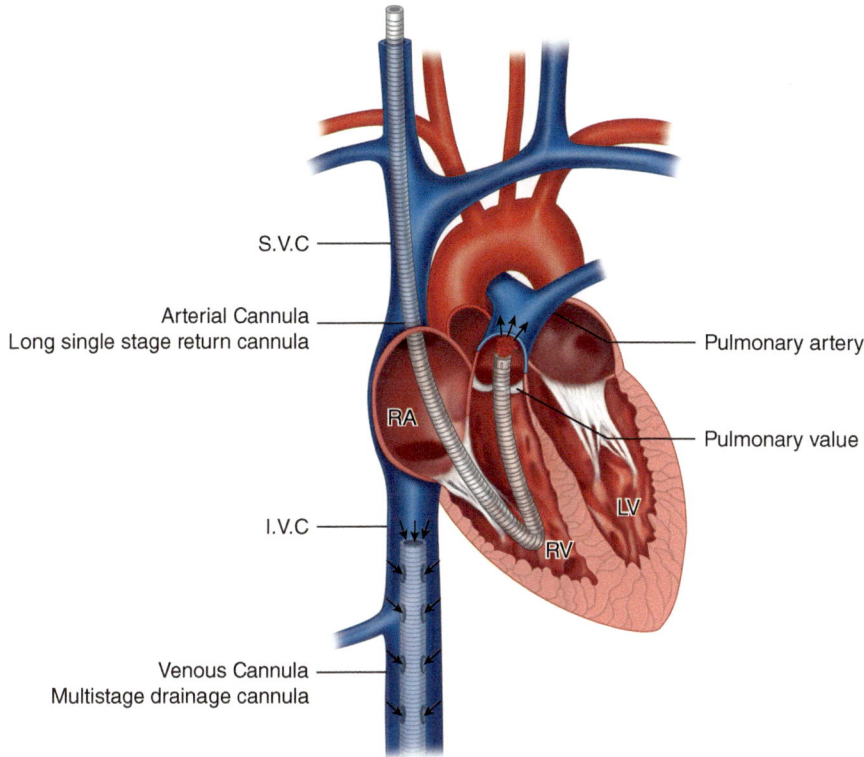

Fig. 7.7 Veno-pulmonary arterial cannulation (VPa)

Peripheral VA ECMO

Fem-Femoral VA ECMO

Femoral cannulation is the most common configuration for VA ECMO. *It is* often an emergent procedure and has been a step forward in the extensive application of VA ECMO everywhere in the hospital and was recently performed also outside the hospital (Fig. 7.8).

In this configuration cannulation, the right femoral vein (RFV) cannulation is usually preferred due to relatively vertical course of the right femoral and common iliac veins into the right-sided inferior vena cava, although it is not always available (i.e., in the case of hematoma, anatomical changes, venous disorders, procedural needs such as trans-septal puncture). The left common iliac vein, on the other hand, crosses the vertebral column and aorta to reach the inferior vena cava, resulting in greater risk from left-sided venous cannulation.

Venous blood drainage is more efficient when a long 55 cm multistage drainage cannula is positioned at the level of SVC-right atrium junction or higher in the SVC as compared to a lower position [4].

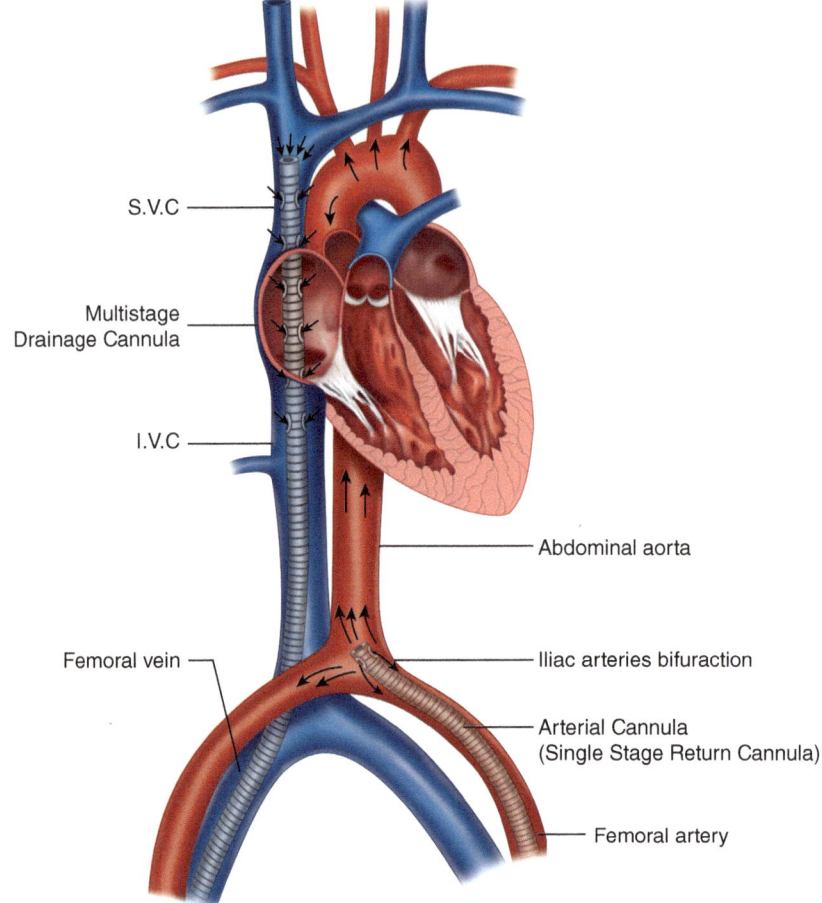

Fig. 7.8 Peripheral VA ECMO

For arterial cannulation, the contralateral side is recommended; however, unilateral cannulation may be unavoidable. Some believe that if a surgical cut-down is mandatory, ipsilateral cannulation should be used, while others prefer contralateral cannulation. They argue that any complication, such as hematoma or infection, will affect both cannulated vessels. An arterial cannula 23 cm long is preferred in this configuration to reach the bifurcation of iliac arteries.

The main *disadvantages* include differential hypoxia, thrombus formation at the aortic root, left ventricular distension, and ischemia in the lower extremities. In addition, patients with significant peripheral vascular disease may not be able to undergo femoral cannulation. This is discussed in the section on complication.

Fem-Subclavian or Fem-Axillary

A VA ECMO cannulation configuration uses the subclavian artery for arterial access and the femoral vein for venous access. The distal right subclavian artery is exposed through a subclavicular incision of 3–4 cm, distal to the thyrocervical trunk branching. After the subclavian artery slings proximally and distally, a graft of 8 mm is sutured from end to end. A 21–24 Fr cannula is tunneled from another incision, inserted into the graft, and advanced to the arteriotomy. Similarly, you can cannulate the axillary artery using the same method [15].

A major *advantage* of this method of cannulation is the fact that it provides antegrade flow to the arterial system. This is similar to central cannulation with reduced afterload on the left ventricle. A further benefit can be gained if the configuration is switched to upper body cannulation by making the venous access through the right IJ vein. By doing this, the lower limbs will be freed up for rehabilitation to take place.

Disadvantage: Similar to a percutaneous approach, the risk of bleeding and infection can be higher with surgery. However, when compared to a similar approach using femoral cannulation, the risk is lower. Aside from that, ECMO cannulation cannot be performed during cardiac arrest since surgery is required, and it has to be performed in an operating room, so it is not feasible during an emergency. The right upper limb may experience swelling due to hyperperfusion, compartmental syndrome, as well as limb ischemia in the same way as femoral cannulation.

Central VA ECMO

Central cannulation is used during postcardiotomy cardiogenic shock. It already employs cannulas as part of a typical cardiopulmonary bypass (CPB). A venous cannula is in the right atrium, and an arterial cannula is in the ascending aorta. The size of the cannulas is defined by body surface area and the calculated extracorporeal flow necessary to achieve the patient's metabolic requirements. Usually, we use 22–24 Fr for aortic cannulation; for venous cannulation, we use a two-stage cannula ranging from 32–34 to 40–46 Fr (Fig. 7.9).

The main advantages of this type of ECLS are efficient venous drainage and typically allowing for more effective cardiac decompression than in peripheral cannulation. The arterial flow returns to the ascending aorta in an antegrade manner with less concern on left ventricular afterload and differential hypoxemia. It also allows complete control over left ventricular decompression by placing a vent, usually via the right superior pulmonary vein. It is of the utmost importance to secure the cannulas in their position; purse-string sutures and tourniquets tied around the cannula is the standard procedure. This is to prevent bleeding from the cannulation site or their displacement during the following care in the ICU.

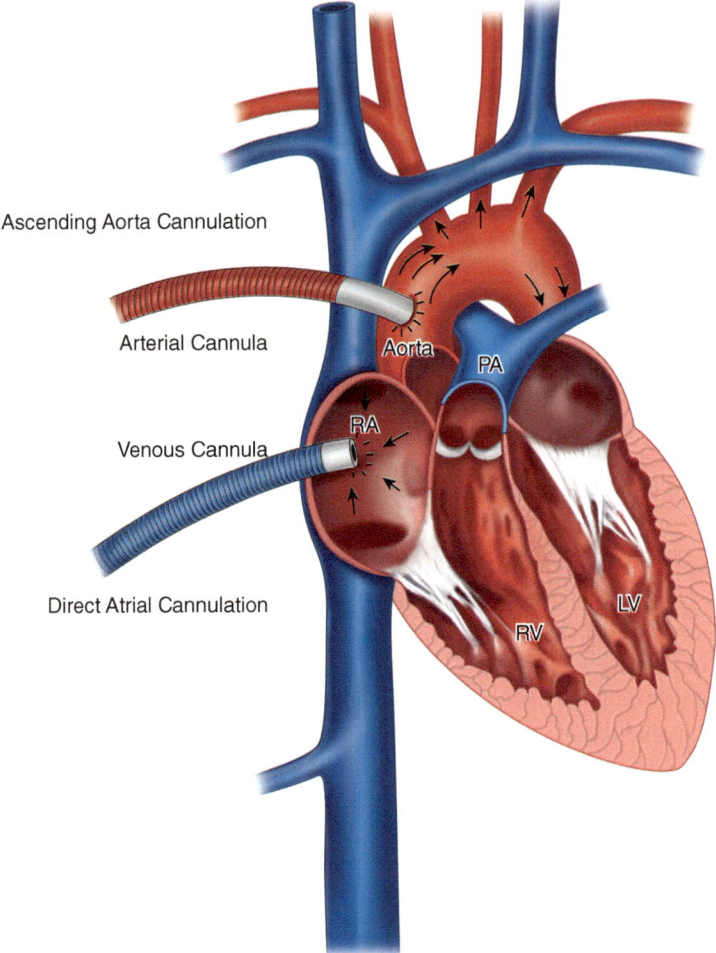

Ascending Aorta Cannulation

Arterial Cannula

Venous Cannula

Direct Atrial Cannulation

Fig. 7.9 Central VA ECMO: drainage cannula into the right atrium—return arterial cannula into the ascending aorta

A key disadvantage of central cannulation is that it requires opening the chest to initiate and discontinue ECMO. As such, central cannulation increases the risk of bleeding, surgical re-exploration, and mediastinitis. Furthermore, central cannulation generally precludes extubation and patient mobilization [5].

Hybrid Configurations

ECLS basic configurations have their own limitations. It is possible that VA ECLS will not be able to provide adequate cardiac and cerebral oxygenation, especially in the case of peripheral cannulation. In the same way, if a patient receiving VV ECLS suffers from decreasing heart function, some form of hemodynamic support may be required. This is where hybrid systems come in. A variety of configurations have been reported in the past few years. In this part, we focus on the most described systems. In the international summary report of ELSO, hybrid ECMO represents approximately 2% of all documented ECMO runs [19].

It is important to note that, according to the ELSO Maastricht Treaty for ECLS Nomenclature published in 2019, there are specific rules defining configurations. We will summarize some of the most important rules here:

An uppercase letter is used for all cannulas contributing to major drainage or return flow. A hyphen in the configuration described indicates the extracorporeal membrane lung (ML). Consequently, when a one-lumen cannula configuration is used, the draining cannula will always be on the left and the return cannula on the right. Hence, the designation ("V-V" or "V-A" cannulation) can be interpreted correctly, with V symbolizing venous, A symbolizing arterial, and-symbolizing ML. In the case of a third (and sometimes a fourth) cannula is placed, the additional uppercase letter is placed on the outer side of the existing cannula. As an example, if a second venous drainage cannula is added, the "V" will be placed outside the first drainage cannula and to the left of the hyphen: "VV-A." In the event that a second reentry cannula is placed in any vein during V-A for improvement of systemic oxygenation in parallel with the initial arterial cannula, the letter V is added to the outer right side of the diagram to represent the return flow (V-AV). As an arterial cannula is added to a "V-V" configuration, the configuration will be expressed as "V-VA" [18].

Veno-Venovenous (VV-V)

A third cannula for drainage can be used in VV ECMO cases with refractory hypoxemia and limited ECMO flow. This will improve ECMO flow while decreasing the risk of hemolysis from high negative pressures on the primary drainage cannulas (Fig. 7.10).

Veno-Arteriovenous Configuration (V-AV)

When VA ECMO does not provide adequate oxygenated blood to the patient's upper body (usually referred to as "Harlequin syndrome" or "North/South syndrome"), an additional inflow cannula can be implanted into the internal jugular vein to deliver oxygenated blood to the pulmonary circulation. By increasing the return of oxygenated blood into the right ventricle and pulmonary circulation, differential hypoxemia can be effectively corrected as oxygenated blood is delivered to the left ventricle through the pulmonary circulation, which then reaches the coronary arteries and aortic arch vessels (Fig. 7.11).

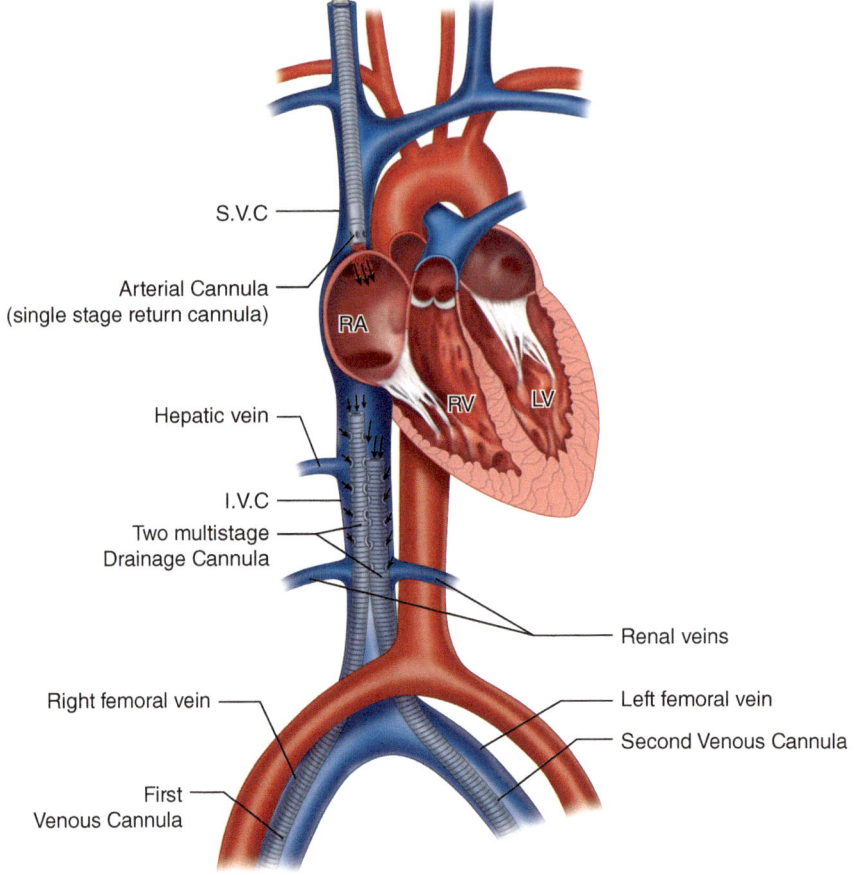

Fig. 7.10 Veno-venovenous (VV-V)

Veno-Venoarterial Cannulation (VV-A)

This is a particular variant of VA ECMO, which utilizes a second venous cannula to improve drainage. When a patient suffers severe left-sided, right-sided, or biventricular heart failure, VA ECMO is intended to support hemodynamics and unload the heart. Some patients, however, do not have adequate venous drainage, which reduces ECMO flow. The cause of this can be related to an insufficient cannula diameter or a very large patient. A third cannula draining from the right atrium is often sufficient to optimize unloading, increase upper body drainage, and minimize intracardiac shunts. Furthermore, VV-A may help restore flow through a draining cannula or reduce hemolysis caused by high flows in patients with insufficient drainage (Fig. 7.12).

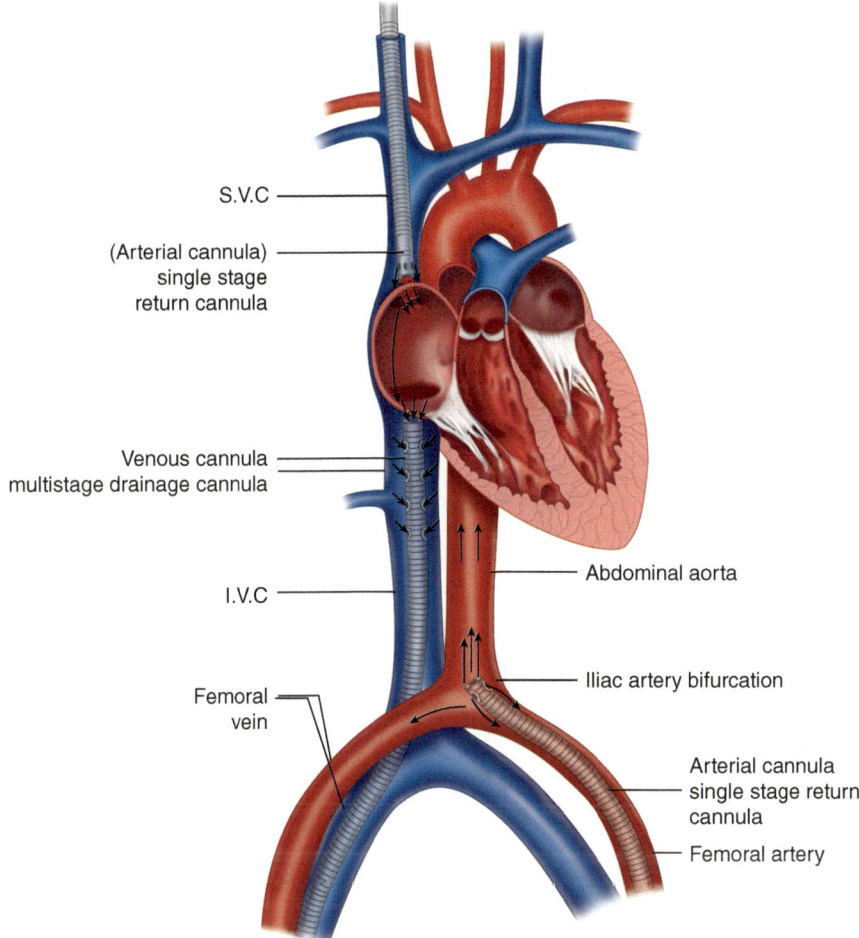

S.V.C

(Arterial cannula)
single stage
return cannula

Venous cannula
multistage drainage cannula

I.V.C

Femoral
vein

Abdominal aorta

Iliac artery bifurcation

Arterial cannula
single stage return
cannula

Femoral artery

Fig. 7.11 This configuration represents veno-arteriovenous configuration (V-AV) and veno-venoarterial cannulation (V-VA)

Veno-Venoarterial Cannulation (V-VA)

A V-VA ECMO is initiated when heart failure develops during a VV ECMO therapy for ARDS. The presence of left-sided heart failure in cases such as septic cardiomy-opathy or myocarditis will make the insufficient cardiac output a significant prob-lem regardless of venous blood oxygenation. The plan is to add a VA ECMO component to the running VV ECMO by introducing a third cannula to supply blood to the aorta. It is imperative to know that V-VA and V-AV are the same can-nulation configuration, but the nomenclature changes according to the primary con-figuration support vs. the later added cannula (Fig. 7.11).

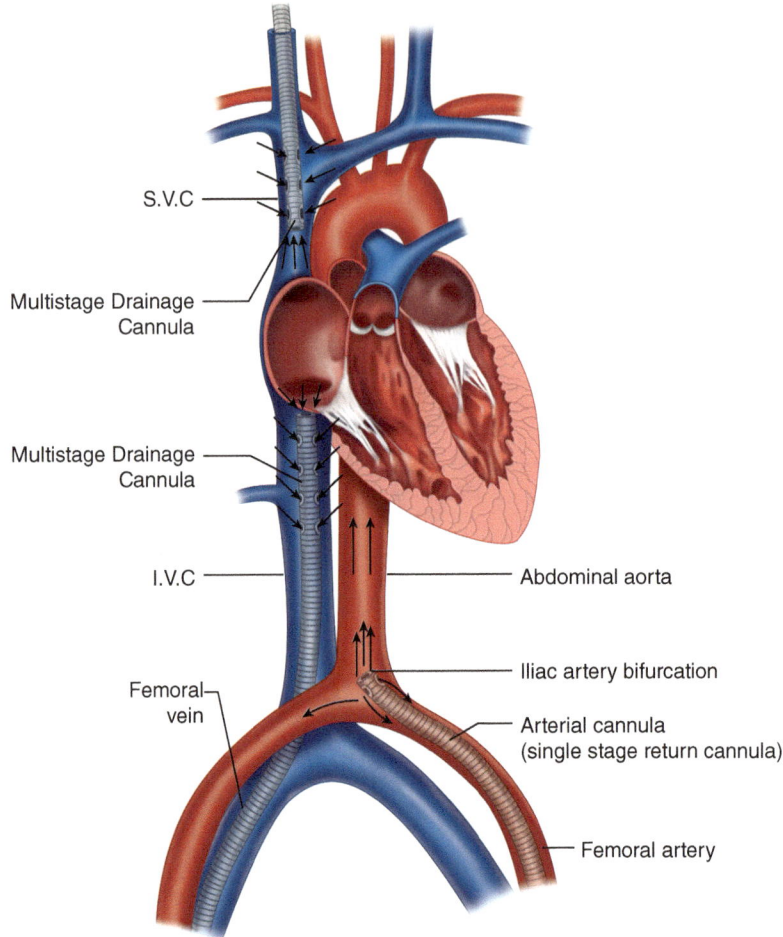

Fig. 7.12 Veno-venoarterial cannulation (VV-A)

In all hybrid configurations, the arterial and venous reinfusion flows are titrated with vascular clamps (Hoffman clamp) (Fig. 7.13) that direct blood flow toward a preferred cannula. When we initiate V-AV or VV-A ECMO, we aim to direct two-thirds of the reinfusion blood flow toward the primary arterial cannula. The flow rate through the secondary added cannula and its tubing should be at least 1 L/min, regardless of the total flow. This is to prevent thrombus formation within the cannula and tubing system. The patient's physiologic needs are then met in a dynamic manner as intrinsic cardiac and pulmonary function improves [17].

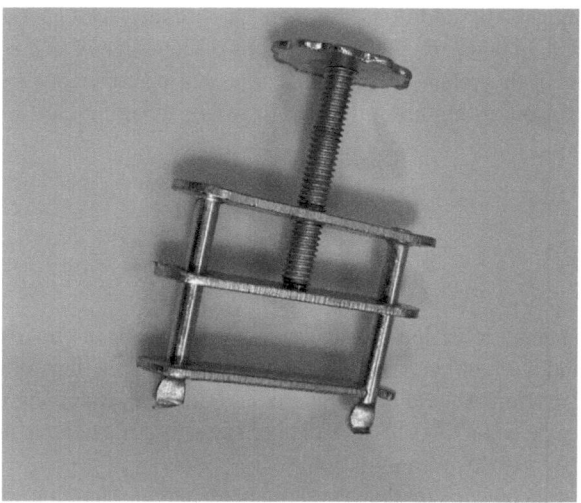

Fig. 7.13 Hoffman clamp

Cannulation Technique

- *Peripheral Cannulation*

  Peripheral cannulation is the mainstay of ECMO, regardless of the disease process or the support method used. It is referred to as puncturing the vessel outside the thoracic or abdominal cavity. Percutaneous cannulation by the Seldinger technique, cut-down cannulation, or a combination of both can be performed (the semi-Seldinger technique). Until the 1990s, the traditional approach to cannulation for ECMO was an open surgical approach; even venous cannulation was primarily achieved by surgical or "open" cut-down procedures, and this approach still remains an important option. This surgical technique allows direct visualization of anatomy, confirming cannula entry into the vessels and securing hemostasis with purse-string sutures. Through time, thin-walled wire-reinforced cannulas were developed, and ultrasound machines became more readily available, enabling the percutaneous technique to spread, and clinicians now can perform cannulation at the patient's bedside instead of moving the patient to the operating room [3].

- *Central Cannulation*

  The term central cannulation refers to any cannulation of the cardiac structure, intrathoracic aorta, or pulmonary artery. These procedures require sternotomies or thoracotomies.

- *Percutaneous Cannulation*

  The percutaneous Seldinger technique is the preferred method of cannulation, and it should be used whenever possible and safely. Cannulas placed percutaneously are likely less susceptible to infectious issues when placed with the appropriate technique. In addition, they are less likely to experience bleeding complications. In addition, the percutaneous placement makes it easier to secure the cannulas so they cannot dislodge. The use of percutaneous cannulation can even be superior to ongoing CPR if ultrasound imaging can provide reliable visualization.

Preparation

1. Cannulation under local anesthesia is possible for a patient who is spontaneously breathing and alert, but generally patients are sedated and intubated.
2. Ultrasound machine should be with vascular linear probe and phased array probe of transthoracic echo TTE. TEE is the gold standard if available and mandatory with dual-lumen bicaval cannulation.
3. Prior to cannula placement, the vessel diameter and its anatomic structure should be examined by duplex sonography whenever possible to determine the site and size of the cannula.
4. Coagulation parameters need to be checked, and packed RBCs need to be prepared.
5. Cannula insertion might increase material consumption, i.e., the need for additional needles, guidewires, and dilator packs.
6. If patients do not receive antibiotics during their procedure, intravenous prophylactic antibiotics can be considered, with an antibiotic choice and schedule based on the institution's guidelines. If prophylactic antibiotics are not required to treat the underlying infection, they should not be continued during ECLS support [12].

General Steps of Cannulation [6]

1. There should be adequate exposure of cannulation site as well as echo or ultrasound examination site for monitoring cannula placement, and it should be performed under complete aseptic techniques.
2. The procedure is best performed by two operators.
3. Upon puncturing the vessel with 5–6 Fr micropuncture or directly with 20-gauge needle under ultrasound guidance, micropuncture with short and soft guidewire is preferred when there is uncertainty of the vessel access. After the first dilator applied, a 100–150 cm soft-tipped but stiff guidewire is advanced.
4. Once the guidewire tip is confirmed in position by echo, a dose of 5000 IU of heparin is injected. Then start to pass the dilators over the guidewire, in a stepwise approach to enlarge the access until the cannula size is achieved. Sometimes, we use the holding introducers available with the cannula for the last step of dilatation. Every time you insert a dilator, check the guidewire

movement across the dilator to make sure that no kinks have happened and the guidewire is freely moving in and out.

5. When the dilator is exchanged, it is crucial to manually compress the puncture site to avoid excessive bleeding. One should not over-dilate to avoid bleeding at the puncture site.

6. If the guidewire does not move freely inside the dilator, retract the dilator proximally and guidewire should be withdrawn a few centimeters to be checked for any kink; if kink is present, try to advance the dilator over the kinked part outside the patient and then continue the dilatation process; otherwise, the guidewire should be replaced.

7. If a guidewire becomes entangled at the abdominal level, there are frequently no other options than to manipulate the wire carefully back and forth. In the operating room or Cath lab, fluoroscopy may be used as well to facilitate wire advancement. However, it should not be forgotten that there are situations where open cannula placement should be preferred [8].

8. When advancing the cannula, ensure that the introducer is beyond the cannula tip by at least a few centimeters. It is extremely important to advance the introducer with the cannula as a single unit.

9. Once the cannula is inserted, the position of the cannula tip should be checked by ultrasound, then remove the guidewire first and then the introducer, and clamp the cannula once you see the blood backflow. Removing the guidewire and the introducer simultaneously may result in excessive bleeding as the introducer is shorter than the guidewire and while blood backflow the guidewire still remaining inside the cannula resulting in more blood loss.

10. The cannula should be fully flushed by saline and connected to the tubing of ECMO system with underwater seal technique. It is important to ensure that the tubing is free of air bubbles.

11 In all configurations and to avoid external bleeding, the cutaneous insertion point of the cannula should be closely tied around the cannula using separated stitches and/or a cutaneous purse-string suture. The cannulas must be secured and fixed to the skin in several points. Cannulas need to be draped, and its insertion point to the skin should be marked according to institution policy.

12. Repeat echocardiography and chest X-ray to confirm the position of the cannulas and screen for any complication.

Special Consideration in Cannulation

- *Percutaneous Cannulation of the Jugular Vein*

    Prior to VV ECMO cannulation scan by ultrasound, usually right internal jugular and both femoral veins are imaged in the supine position, but if the internal jugular vein is not distended from the positive intrathoracic pressure accompanying mechanical ventilation, the patient is placed in Trendelenburg position.

Special attention should be paid that guidewire advance is guided either by echo or by fluoroscopy to ensure that the wire traverses through IVC to avoid injury or coiling in the RT atrium or RT ventricle.

- *Dual-lumen bicaval cannula insertion*: The guidewire is advanced under fluoroscopic imaging or TEE through the intrahepatic inferior vena cava to the level of the iliac bifurcation to ensure inadvertent cannulation of the hepatic vein and prevent accidental dislodgment of the wire during cannulation.

  Transesophageal echocardiography is used to confirm the reinfusion jet across the tricuspid valve. Radiopaque markers on some of the commercially available cannula's drainage and reinfusion ports aid in the initial placement and subsequent maintenance of the catheter's appropriate orientation during the patient's management course.

- *Percutaneous Cannulation of the Femoral Artery*

  It is mandatory to assess the size of the artery by ultrasound to select the cannula size; a bigger cannula most likely will take the whole artery diameter causing distal limb ischemia. A single stick to the artery is preferred, and the longitudinal approach by ultrasound will help to avoid transfixion of the artery.

  If puncture is not successful or if the guidewire gets caught and there is no alternative access site, surgical exploration of the access vessels is warranted. Moreover, where the caliber of the vessels is unusually small, percutaneous cannula placement is hazardous. In these cases, suturing a Dacron graft with a diameter of 6–8 mm to the arterial vessel is the best choice.

- *Percutaneous Cannulation of the Distal Perfusion Cannula*

  It is also recommended to implement distal limb perfusion cannula with a 6–9 Fr vascular reinforced sheath instead of a standard access cannula as it prevents kinking. It is favorable to place a wire distally prior to placement of the actual arterial cannula, since distal flow is usually considerably lower after placement of the arterial cannula. However, during an emergency situation or in case of patients with ECPR, this can be done later after the femoral artery cannulation. The bifurcation of the common femoral artery is located by ultrasound. In an antegrade manner, the superficial femoral artery (SFA) is accessed just past the bifurcation. Ensure that the wire can pass freely down the leg. This can be guided by fluoroscopy, but it is not usually necessary. Afterward, the SFA is cannulated with the sheath. Later, a high-pressure tube will be used to connect this sheath to the Luer Lock port on the arterial cannula to allow circuit blood to perfuse the lower limbs. DPC may be inserted antegrade as the case with SFA cannulation or retrograde if posterior tibial or dorsalis pedis was cannulated [2].

- *Surgical Cut-Down Cannulation*

  The open approach typically involves surgical exposure of the vessel with large incision, placement of ligatures, venotomy (or arteriotomy), insertion of the cannula (with or without a blunt loading dilator), ligation of the vessel distal to and around the cannula, or preferably placement of an end-to-side graft to the artery with insertion of the cannula into the graft with ligation and closure of the incision. The advantages of the open approach include the ability to properly size the cannula and ensure intraluminal placement while monitoring to avoid vessel injury. The disadvantages include the increased risk for surgical site bleeding, need for surgical repair for decannulation, and obstruction of the vessel if ligation is required. The latter can be avoided if an end-to-side graft was done [7].

• *Modified Seldinger (Hybrid Technique)*

A large or smaller incision is made in this technique to expose the vessels, followed by a needle puncture distally to the incision, which creates a tract for percutaneous insertion. The access into the vessel is performed visually, and the skin and subcutaneous tissue are closed, preventing vessel ligation and incisions, as well as closing the skin without removing the cannula through an incision, reducing bleeding risks.

Complications of Cannulation

Vascular Injury

Vascular injury can affect the target or adjacent vessels, resulting in dissection, pseudoaneurysm, and retroperitoneal bleeding. The injury usually occurs during cannulation or cannula removal. If the injury occurs during cannulation, it may result in vascular access being unavailable. Attempting surgical repair and completing the cannulation immediately are imperative; otherwise, failure is likely.

An access-site pseudoaneurysm can be suspected by painful pulsatile swelling and can be confirmed by ultrasound. Therefore, early recognition of such complications is vital to initiating treatment as soon as possible. If untreated, access-site pseudoaneurysms can result in serious complications, including arterial occlusion, rupture, or hematoma, and lead to infection. Access-site pseudoaneurysms can be treated immediately with local compression. Surgery is required if the pseudoaneurysm is large and/or associated with other complications. Endovascular treatment is an alternative to surgical repair for small pseudoaneurysms or those unsuitable for surgery.

The majority of arterial dissections are asymptomatic. Dissection-induced arterial occlusion must be differentiated from thromboembolic occlusion. In most cases, the arterial cannula is relocated to a different location, and a stent is inserted to treat dissection symptoms.

Further, the presence of anticoagulation can worsen the complications if not detected early. As a result, large internal hematomas can develop from minor vascular injuries. Hemodynamic changes and decreased hematocrit make such vascular injuries suspectable, and imaging can confirm them. The patients are managed by correcting their anticoagulation and receiving transfusions. Endovascular embolization may be necessary if conservative measures do not resolve the problem. There are very few cases when open surgery is required [16].

Leg Ischemia

Ischemia of the lower limb is one of the major risks associated with cannulation of the femoral artery. It can also happen to upper limbs in case of axillary and subclavian cannulation. If limb ischemia is not detected in time, sufficient muscle necrosis can occur that may require fasciotomy or even amputation. Careful clinical examination, Doppler monitoring of distal pulses, and plethysmography assessment with pulse oximetry can help identify this condition early. Another important tool to monitor distal leg perfusion, near-infrared spectroscopy (NIRS), is very useful. It is important to obtain baseline values on both legs prior to cannulation to be able to validate leg ischemia. As mentioned before, DPC cannulation with different approaches can mitigate this risk.

An end-to-side graft can be applied and cannulated as an alternative to arterial cannulation for the femoral artery or the subclavian artery. In this way, a large cannula can be used for optimal blood flow, avoiding obstructions and distal ischemia. In addition, the grafting approach may be better suited to long-term venoarterial support.

Lower Limb DVT

Deep venous thrombosis can occur if the femoral vein drainage cannula occupies the entire vein.

Compartmental Syndrome

Hyperperfusion states can result in swollen and hyperemic limb in arterial cannulation in some cases where the axillary or subclavian artery was cannulated, or if the femoral artery and vein are cannulated on the ipsilateral side. The presence of arterial or venous outflow obstruction, in addition to hyperperfusion, can make compartmental syndrome a serious condition in which high compartment pressure may lead to limb ischemia. Management in these cases involves addressing each cause and may include relocating the cannulation site. In some patients, a fasciotomy is required [9].

Bleeding

Among all bleeding complications, cannulation sites are the most common source of bleeding. Although most cases are minimal, intervention is sometimes required. As a first step, it is important to verify adequate levels of anticoagulation, adequate platelet counts, and a normal prothrombin time as well as adequate fibrinogen levels. Anticoagulation targets can be reduced, and topical hemostatic agents can be applied. Avoiding large incisions and over-dilatation during cannula insertion can minimize bleeding by fitting the cannula tightly. Surgical cannulation may require re-exploration if more conservative measures fail.

Infection

Extracorporeal support patients may face infection problems at the site of cannulation, and groin infections are particularly likely to occur in obese and malnourished patients. To prevent infection, it is essential to use a strict aseptic technique when placing the cannula and when handling it afterward. A cannula infection is detected when there is cellulitis, swelling, or discharge around the cannula. Antibiotic treatment should be initiated as soon as an infection is detected, as well as surgical intervention if necessary. When bacteremia persists after treatment with antibiotics, replacing the extracorporeal circuit may be necessary as seeding of the large surface area circuit might prevent the eradication of infection.

Even though recannulation at a different site is risky and challenging, it may be necessary if antimicrobials and changing the extracorporeal circuit fail to treat cannula-site infections [13].

Configuration Complication

Differential Hypoxia

In peripherally cannulated VA ECMO patients with concomitant lung failure or ventilator mismanagement, the Harlequin, or North South, syndrome occurs due to differential hypoxemia between the upper and lower body. It results when retrograde oxygenated blood from the femoral arterial cannula meets undrained blood from the RA, which traverses the pulmonary vasculature and leaves the left ventricle (LV). As a result of low oxygenation in the blood ejected from the LV, coronary arteries and cerebral circulation may be malperfused. This is determined by native lung function, volume status, and cardiac function.

A persistent dual-circuit circulation is likely to result from this watershed. As a result, the upper body is perfused with poorly oxygenated blood that travels from the heart to the superior vena cava (SVC) and back to the heart without entering the ECMO circuit, and the ECMO circuit supplies well-oxygenated blood to the lower body, which returns to the ECMO circuit via the IVC.

Right Ventricular Rupture

Right ventricular rupture and tamponade may complicate right IJ vein cannulation. The guidewire can damage the right ventricle, as can dilators or the cannula. This is a major complication that requires urgent surgical intervention if it occurs. To avoid this, cannulation must be done with extreme caution and under the guidance of TEE or fluoroscopy [14].

References

1. Javidfar J, Brodie D, Wang D, Ibrahimiye AN, Yang J, Zwischenberger JB, Sonett J, Bacchetta M. Use of bicaval dual-lumen catheter for adult venovenous extracorporeal membrane oxygenation. Ann Thorac Surg. 2011;91:1763–9.
2. Ramaiah C, Babu A. ECMO cannulation techniques. In: Firstenberg M, editor. Extracorporeal membrane oxygenation: advances in therapy. London: IntechOpen; 2016. https://doi.org/10.5772/64338.
3. Pavlushkov E, Berman M, Valchanov K. Cannulation techniques for extracorporeal life support. Ann Transl Med. 2017;5(4):70. https://doi.org/10.21037/atm.2016.11.47. PMID: 28275615; PMCID: PMC5337209.
4. Ruggeri L, Evangelista M, Consolo F, et al. Peripheral VA-ECMO venous cannulation: which side for the femoral cannula? Intensive Care Med. 2017;43:468–9. https://doi.org/10.1007/s00134-016-4636-5.
5. Jayaraman AL, Cormican D, Shah P, Ramakrishna H. Cannulation strategies in adult veno-arterial and veno-venous extracorporeal membrane oxygenation: techniques, limitations, and special considerations. Ann Card Anaesth. 2017;20(Supplement):S11–8. https://doi.org/10.4103/0971-9784.197791. PMID: 28074818; PMCID: PMC5299823.
6. Keyser A, Philipp A, Zeman F, Lubnow M, Lunz D, Zimmermann M, Schmid C. Percutaneous cannulation for extracorporeal life support in severely and morbidly obese patients. J Intensive Care Med. 2020;35(9):919–26. https://doi.org/10.1177/0885066618801547. Epub 2018 Sep 19. PMID: 30231666.
7. Conrad SA, Grier LR, Scott LK, Green R, Jordan MRN. Percutaneous cannulation for extracorporeal membrane oxygenation by intensivists: a retrospective single-institution case series. Crit Care Med. 2015;43(5):1010–5. https://doi.org/10.1097/CCM.0000000000000883.
8. Ganslmeier P, Philipp A, Rupprecht L, Diez C, Arlt M, Mueller T, Pfister K, Hilker M, Schmid C. Percutaneous cannulation for extracorporeal life support. Thorac Cardiovasc Surg. 2011;59(2):103–7. https://doi.org/10.1055/s-0030-1250635. Epub 2011 Mar 7. PMID: 21384306.
9. Chamogeorgakis T, Lima B, Shafii AE, Nagpal D, Pokersnik JA, Navia JL, Mason D, Gonzalez-Stawinski GV. Outcomes of axillary artery side graft cannulation for extracorporeal membrane oxygenation. J Thorac Cardiovasc Surg. 2013;145(4):1088–92. https://doi.org/10.1016/j.jtcvs.2012.08.070. Epub 2012 Sep 20. PMID: 22999514.
10. Abrams D, Brodie D, Javidfar J, Brenner K, Wang D, Zwischenberger J, et al. Insertion of bicaval dual-lumen cannula via the left internal jugular vein for extracorporeal membrane oxygenation. ASAIO J. 2012;58:636–7.
11. Shafii AE, McCurry KR. Subclavian insertion of the bicaval dual lumen cannula for venovenous extracorporeal membrane oxygenation. Ann Thorac Surg. 2012;94:663–5.
12. Extracorporeal life support organization task force on infections. Infection control and extracorporeal life support 2010. http://elso.org/downloads/resources/committees/infectiousdisease-and-antibiotic/Infection-Control-and-Extracorporeal-Life-Support.pdf.

13. Bizzarro MJ, Conrad SA, Kaufman DA, Rycus P. Extracorporeal life support organization task force on infections, extracorporeal membrane oxygenation. Infections acquired during extracorporeal membrane oxygenation in neonates, children, and adults. Pediatr Crit Care Med. 2011;12(3):277–81. https://doi.org/10.1097/PCC.0b013e3181e28894. PMID: 20495508.
14. Hirose H, Yamane K, Marhefka G, et al. Right ventricular rupture and tamponade caused by malposition of the Avalon cannula for venovenous extracorporeal membrane oxygenation. J Cardiothorac Surg. 2012;7:36. https://doi.org/10.1186/1749-8090-7-36.
15. Javidfar J, Brodie D, Costa J, Miller J, Jurrado J, LaVelle M, Newmark A, Takayama H, Sonett JR, Bacchetta M, et al. ASAIO J. 2012;58(5):494–8. https://doi.org/10.1097/MAT.0b013e318268ea15.
16. Pillai AK, Bhatti Z, Bosserman AJ, Mathew MC, Vaidehi K, Kalva SP. Management of vascular complications of extra-corporeal membrane oxygenation. Cardiovasc Diagn Ther. 2018;8(3):372–7. https://doi.org/10.21037/cdt.2018.01.11. PMID: 30057883; PMCID: PMC6039794.
17. Biscotti M, Lee A, Basner RC, Agerstrand C, Abrams D, Brodie D, Bacchetta M. Hybrid configurations via percutaneous access for extracorporeal membrane oxygenation: a single centre experience. ASAIO J. 2014;60:635–42.
18. Broman LM, Taccone FS, Lorusso R, Malfertheiner MV, Pappalardo F, Di Nardo M, Belliato M, Bembea MM, Barbaro RP, Diaz R, Grazioli L, Pellegrino V, Mendonca MH, Brodie D, Fan E, Bartlett RH, McMullan MM, Conrad SA. The ELSO Maastricht treaty for ECLS nomenclature: abbreviations for cannulation configuration in extracorporeal life support – a position paper of the extracorporeal life support organization. Crit Care. 2019;23(1):36. https://doi.org/10.1186/s13054-019-2334-8. PMID: 30736845; PMCID: PMC6367794.
19. Ius F, Sommer W, Tudorache I, Avsar M, Siemeni T, Salman J, Puntigam J, Optenhoefel J, Greer M, Welte T, Wiesner O, Haverich A, Hoeper M, Keuhn C, Warnecke G. Veno-veno-arterial extracorporeal membrane oxygenation for respiratory failure with severe hemodynamic impairment: technique and early outcome. Interact Cardiovasc Thorac Surg. 2015;20:761–7.

Chapter 8
Complications and Emergencies Associated with ECMO

M. Christina Creel-Bulos and Casey Frost Miller

Background and Introduction

ECMO is an exceptionally complex, advanced form of extracorporeal life support that can be associated with various management complications and some may result in emergent situations. Risk for therapy-associated complications should be carefully considered prior to initiation of ECMO, and judicious monitoring for potential complications should continue throughout the duration of ECMO support [1]. The most commonly occurring universal complications associated with any form of ECMO support include bleeding, infection, thrombosis, flow interruptions, and hypoxia [1, 2]. Other complications, such as recirculation and North-South Syndrome, are dependent on the type of ECMO and cannulation strategy used to provide ECMO support (*reference* Fig. 8.1). Most complications occur at any point in time throughout the duration of ECMO therapy, while others are more prone to occur earlier or later in a patient's clinical course (*reference* Fig. 8.2).

There are several emergencies specific to ECMO therapy that all providers caring for patients on this support should not only be aware of, but prepared to manage. The predominance of these emergencies can occur in patients receiving any form of ECMO support and with the exception of a few can be managed similarly. Those

M. C. Creel-Bulos (✉)
Department of Critical Care Medicine, Emory University School of Medicine,
Atlanta, GA, USA

Department of Emergency Medicine, Grady Memoral Hospital, Atlanta, GA, USA
e-mail: maria.christina.creel-bulos@emory.edu

C. F. Miller
Department of Cardiothoracic Surgery, Emory University Hospital,
Atlanta, GA, USA
e-mail: casey.milller@emoryhealthcare.org

© The Author(s), under exclusive license to Springer Nature
Switzerland AG 2024
A. R. Taha et al. (eds.), *ECMO: A Practical Guide to Management*,
https://doi.org/10.1007/978-3-031-59634-6_8

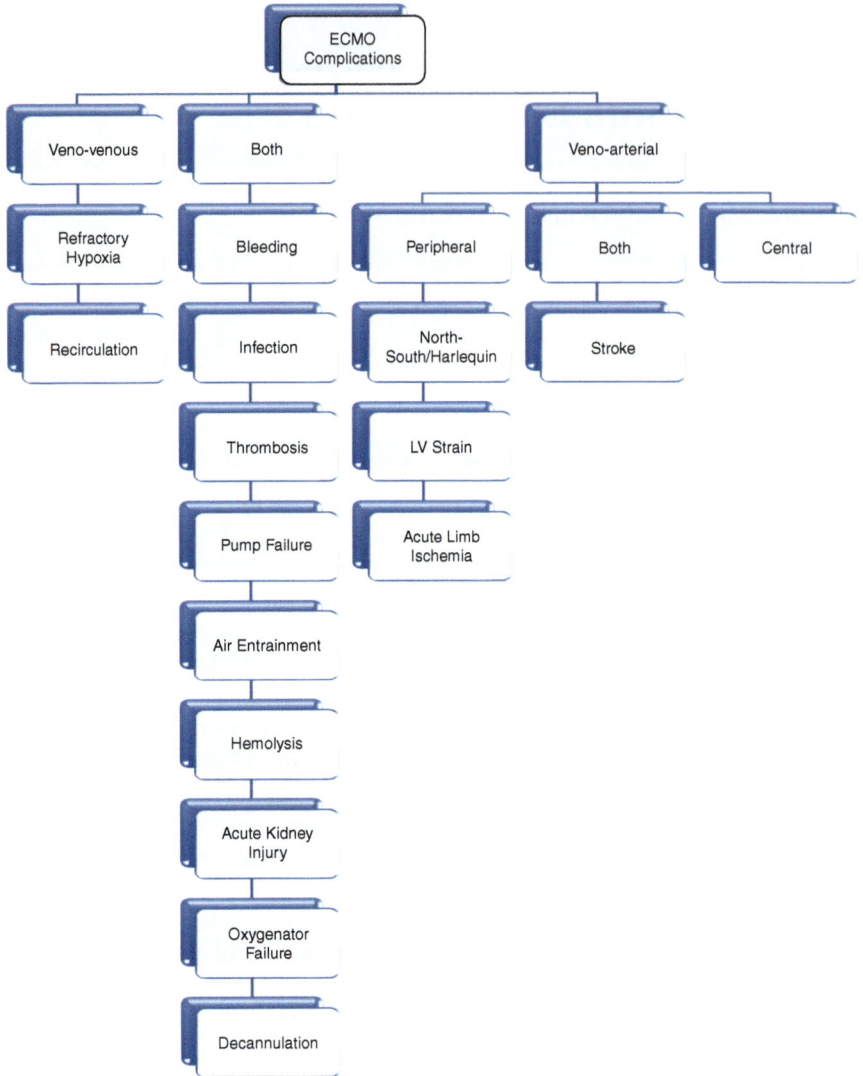

Fig. 8.1 Complications specific to VA ECMO, VV ECMO, or both methods of ECMO

that must be managed specifically based on the form of ECMO support they are receiving are discussed separately.

In this chapter, we will focus on common complications and emergencies that can be experienced while a patient is receiving extracorporeal life support. Specifically, we will address incidence, discuss detection, and briefly mention management of complications and emergencies, respectively.

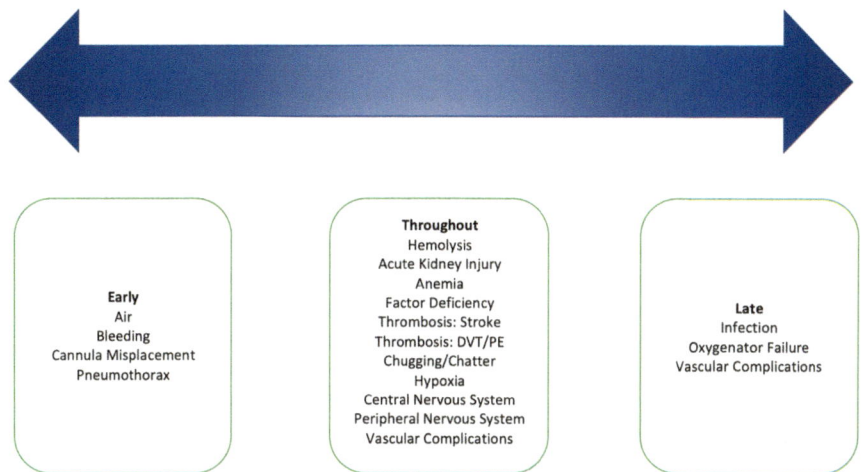

Fig. 8.2 ECMO complications throughout duration of support

Common Complications Associated with ECMO Support

Bleeding

Bleeding is one of the most commonly experienced complications associated with ECMO support. It can occur as frequently as 30–50% in patients receiving this therapy [3]. The degree, location, and source of bleeding are affected by the type of ECMO support being provided, associated cannulation strategy being utilized, as well as the presence of anticoagulation used and associated therapy goals. Comorbid conditions, recent procedures, systemic disease, and coexisting pathology (such as thrombocytopenia, qualitative platelet dysfunction, acquired coagulopathy, or factor deficiencies) can also significantly affect propensity for bleeding.

Bleeding can occur at surgical and/or cannulation sites or anywhere in the body including but not limited to subcutaneous, intramuscular, intrathoracic, intraabdominal, or retroperitoneal spaces. Management of bleeding is dependent on location and degree of bleeding. Non-surgical management options include primary repair or reinforcement with sutures, electrocauterization, and/or application of thrombotic agents. Bleeding can commonly mandate temporary cessation of anticoagulation therapy until hemostasis or source control has been achieved. Often gradual reintroduction of therapy is well tolerated after hemostasis has been achieved, but in other cases, modification of therapeutic goals may be needed or resumption of therapy may be precluded [1, 4]. In severe cases of large volume bleeding, persistent or arterial bleeding, surgical exploration, and/or intervention may be required [5, 6]. Incidence and frequency of bleeding can vary based on multiple factors. Aubron et al. reported up to 34% of patients receiving VA ECMO required surgical exploration for bleeding compared with 17% of patients on VV ECMO [7].

Thrombosis

Thrombosis or the formation of a blood clot within a cardiovascular structure can occur in any region of the body while a patient is receiving ECMO [8]. Not dissimilar to other clinical situations or pathology, thromboembolism can result from prolonged immobility, vascular injury, or hypercoagulability. In this patient subset, it can occur anywhere within the body (i.e., regional to ECMO cannula placement or anywhere systemically) or outside the body in which case the ability to provide ECMO can be compromised. Examples of regional or systemic thromboembolic include but are not limited to deep vein thrombosis with or without pulmonary embolism, systemic thromboembolism and organ ischemia or infarction, left ventricular thrombus, or stroke. Extracorporeal thrombosis can result in pump and oxygenator failure if the development of this goes undetected [9].

The incidence of systemic thrombosis is between 9% and 13% of patients receiving ECMO, whereas "provoked" DVT regional to venous cannulation site can occur in as frequent as 70% of cases [4]. Management can be as simple as reinitiation of anticoagulation therapy, modification of therapeutic goals, increasing dosage of anticoagulation, or utilization of an alternative agent for anticoagulation [10]. In cases in which heparin therapy is utilized, consideration of heparin induced thrombocytopenia (HIT) should be given. Risk assessment and management is consistent with standard critical care practice guidelines that should HIT be diagnosed. Depending on location and severity of thrombosis, thrombolytic therapy, procedural or surgical thromboendarterectomy may be required.

Infection

Not dissimilar to thrombosis, infection can plague patients receiving ECMO either regionally or systemically. The overall incidence of infection is about 10–12% in this patient population [11]. The most commonly reported pathogens identified in patients receiving ECMO support include organisms such as coagulase-negative staphylococci, Candida species, Enterobacteriaceae, and Pseudomonas aeruginosa [11]. If a regional infection limited to superficial skin or connective tissue occurs, it can generally be managed with antibiotic therapy. Should this become more complicated such as developing a fluid collection or abscess, incision and drainage, or even reconfiguration with cannula position change may need to be pursued.

More complicated infections such as thrombophlebitis, mediastinitis, or bloodstream infections can present additional challenges in management; particularly in patients bridging from ECMO to transplantation. Bloodstream infections can be further confounded as they can seed the ECMO membrane or circuit. The incidence of infection has been demonstrated to increase directly in proportion to duration of ECMO support provision [12]. The severity of a patient's critical illness and degree immunocompromise can be influential and should be considered. Other critical illness-related infections (such as ventilator associated pneumonia, gut transloca-tion, and line-associated infections) and nosocomial infections can additionally affect this patient population [12]. These present typically and are not managed differently in patients undergoing ECMO support; although, it is important to note the potential for changes in pharmacokinetics with respect to antimicrobial therapy [13, 14].

Chugging/Chatter

Inadequate drainage can result in interruption of ECMO flow that is commonly termed "chugging" or "chatter." This phenomenon can be associated with hemody-namic instability in venoarterial support or hypoxia resulting in hemodynamic instability for those receiving venovenous ECMO support. Chugging or chatter can be the result of multiple intravascular and extravascular conditions. Some include the following: volume depletion, vessel size and diameter, improper cannula place-ment, or inappropriate cannula size [15]. Management of these complications is centered around the basic principles of temporarily decreasing ECMO flows until consistent flow can be achieved while addressing potential etiologies above with actions such as volume administration, repositioning of patient or cannula, and/or cannula exchange or overall modification ECMO cannulation strategy.

Hypoxia

Impairments in gas exchange associated with either type of respiratory failure can be supported with extracorporeal support. The primary etiology of organ dysfunc-tion and degree of support requirements influence the form of ECMO required. In the case of isolated respiratory failure, venovenous ECMO is traditionally used to correct hypoxic, hypercapnic, or combined respiratory failure. In cases of cardio-genic shock with associated impairments in gas exchange, venoarterial ECMO can additionally aid in gas exchange. On rare occasions, advanced configurations or combinations of ECMO may be required beyond traditional venovenous and/or venoarterial ECMO to support metabolic and systemic demands [16].

The management of hypoxia can be challenging at times and should be executed in a systematic approach that is tailored based on the type of ECMO therapy a patient is receiving.

Refractory hypoxia while a patient is receiving VV ECMO can be attributed to external issues (i.e., equipment malfunction or misuse) or internal physiological needs (i.e., pathological supply and demand mismatch).

The first step in evaluating a patient with refractory hypoxia should be to evalu-ate that there is color change between the drainage and return limbs of the ECMO circuit. This can be done with a visual inspection to ensure the drainage is dark (i.e., deoxygenated) blood relative to return cannula with bright red (i.e., oxygenated) blood. If both limbs are dark, this could mean an issue with the sweep gas or the oxygenator membrane. The oxygen supply to the membrane should be immediately tested to ensure that it is functioning and that it is indeed circulating properly. The oxygen line should be checked for obstruction and to ensure no other medical equipment is blocking the passage of this gas. If oxygen is flowing appropriately, the membrane should be evaluated next.

Hemolysis with subsequent thrombus formation can affect the efficiency of the oxygenator membrane component of ECMO circuit. Membrane health should be evaluated regularly and can be done in numerous ways. Visualization of the membrane can be performed to check for gross evidence of fibrin deposition and/or clot formation. Sufficient accumulation of this can impair gas exchange by way of reducing the relative surface area of the ECMO oxygenator membrane available for efficient gas exchange. Some ECMO consoles allow for pressure monitoring including the ability to continuously visualize pre membrane, post membrane, and delta pressure differences across the membrane. Familiarity with a patient's baseline pressure values and monitoring overall trends in these values can be immensely helpful in detecting oxygenator malfunction in a timely manner prior to patients' overall gas exchange being compromised. Obtaining a post oxygenator blood gas analysis may also provide helpful information when assessing oxygenator health. This can be obtained serially with a regularly scheduled frequency or on an as needed basis. It is important to note that unless access to obtain these samples has been placed prior to initiation of ECMO support, it will require a transient modification in support. Should this access be placed prior to commencement of support and remain in place throughout the duration of support, maintenance will be required to ensure patency. Various serum markers can be utilized to evaluate for the presence of hemolysis and thrombosis, these include but are not limited to LDH, haptoglobin, and plasma free hemoglobin [17, 18].

In the patient receiving venovenous ECMO therapy, refractory hypoxia can be attributed to unique phenomena associated with cannula placement and termed "recirculation" may occur. Evidence of this phenomena can be noted upon evaluating color change between both limbs of the ECMO circuit; specifically, when both are noted to contain bright red oxygenated blood or an intermittent pulsation of bright, oxygenated blood is noted in the drainage component of circuit. Recirculation of oxygenated blood occurs when ECMO drainage and return cannulas are placed too close together resulting in the uptake of oxygenated blood (from the outflow or return cannula) into the drainage or inflow limb of circuit and complete bypass of systemic distribution of oxygenated blood [19, 20]. Radiologic evaluation of cannula placement can be additionally helpful in diagnosing this problem. Ideally, the drainage and return cannulae should have sufficient distance between them to prevent recirculation from occurring.

In patients receiving VA ECMO support via a peripheral cannulation strategy who have sustained significant insult and resultant impairment in gas exchange, refractory hypoxia can indicate the presence of another unique phenomenon termed "North South syndrome" [21]. With the return of native cardiac function, and resultant increase in blood flow through traditional anatomical pathways (i.e., routing through damaged and/or pathologically compromised lung parenchyma), hypoxia can be observed. This can be managed in a variety of ways depending on etiology of respiratory compromise, when recovery is anticipated, estimated duration of VA ECMO support required and/or vascular access limitations. Options include increasing ECMO flows or placement of another venous return limb and conversion to VAV (veno arteriovenous) ECMO. The danger in this phenomenon occurring undetected is that it can result in differential (most commonly cerebral) hypoxia depending on where deoxygenated and oxygenated blood mix and are distributed along the aorta. The only method by which occult cerebral hypoxia can be detected is by way of obtaining blood gas analysis or pulse oximetry from the right upper extremity or forehead. This highlights the importance of ensuring continuous monitoring of oxygen saturation and blood gas monitoring from the right upper extremity in patients who are on VA ECMO support.

While mechanical causes of refractory hypoxia may be easy to assess and diagnose, physiological causes may be more challenging. Any condition resulting in a relative mismatch in the consumption, supply, demand, or deficit in the supply of oxygen can result in refractory hypoxia regardless of the form of ECMO support being utilized to support a patient. Things such as liberation from analgosedation, agitation, fever, shivering, infection or sepsis, tachycardia, and high cardiac output states are commonly encountered etiologies for which each must be individually managed [22].

Other Complications Associated with ECMO Support

There are many other complications associated with utilization of advanced therapies such as ECMO and potential implications on many organ systems within the human body. A brief overview of some of these can be visualized (*Reference* Fig. 8.3) and will be briefly discussed in subsequent sections.

Neurologic Complications

There are various insults that can occur to both the central and peripheral components of the neurological system as a result of ECMO therapy [23]. Cannulation and extended utilization of therapy can result in direct damage or indirect compression of peripheral nerves resulting in neuropraxia or more severe nerve injury. The central nervous system can be compromised by any form of ECMO therapy used as a result of refractory hypoxia or hemorrhage in the setting of anticoagulation therapy. In the setting of VA ECMO or previously unknown and undetected atrial septal defect or PFO, ischemic stroke can additionally occur.

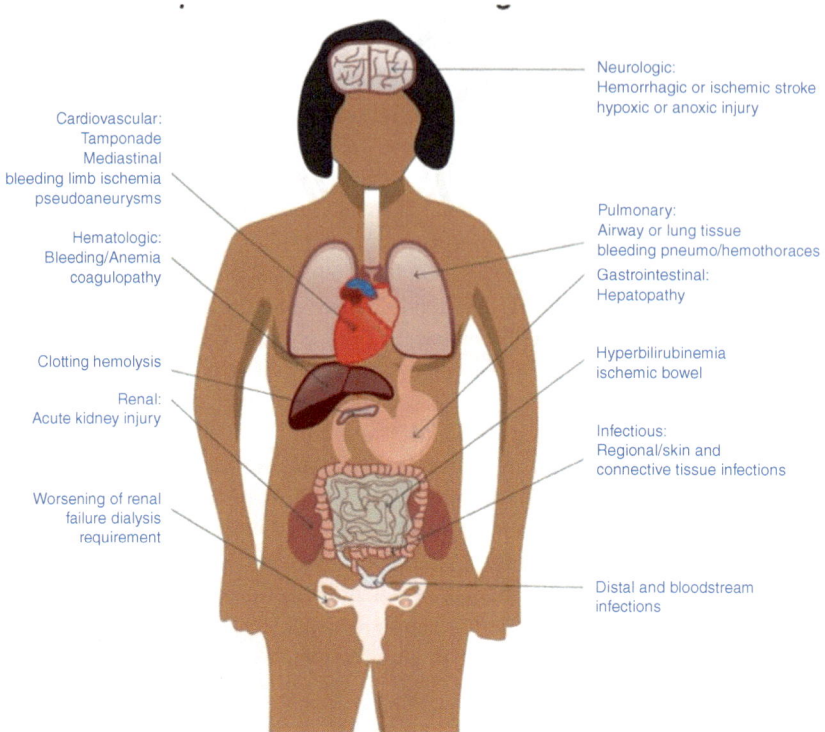

Cardiovascular:
Tamponade
Mediastinal
bleeding limb ischemia
pseudoaneurysms

Hematologic:
Bleeding/Anemia
coagulopathy

Clotting hemolysis

Renal:
Acute kidney injury

Worsening of renal
failure dialysis
requirement

Neurologic:
Hemorrhagic or ischemic stroke
hypoxic or anoxic injury

Pulmonary:
Airway or lung tissue
bleeding pneumo/hemothoraces

Gastrointestinal:
Hepatopathy

Hyperbilirubinemia
ischemic bowel

Infectious:
Regional/skin and
connective tissue infections

Distal and bloodstream
infections

Fig. 8.3 Complications associated with ECMO support by organ system

Pulmonary Complications

Complications resulting from direct injury to the parenchyma of the lung as a result of ECMO therapy are relatively uncommon. On rare occasions, a hemothorax, pneumothorax, or direct injury of parenchyma can occur during cannulation [24]. Pulmonary or alveolar hemorrhage can additionally occur in the setting of anticoagulation. Disease and/or pathology prompting the need for ECMO therapy can result in various secondary complications [24].

Cardiovascular Complications

Cardiovascular complications associated with ECMO therapy are dependent on underlying pathology prompting need for ECMO support or are directly associated with the form of ECMO support and cannulation strategy utilized to provide this support [25]. All patients can develop hematomas related to complicated vascular access and in the setting of anticoagulation. These can occur in many different levels of integument or body cavities. Patients that are cannulated centrally remain at higher risk for mediastinal bleeding and/or development of tamponade. Those receiving peripheral VA ECMO support are at high risk for early development of limb ischemia due to relative redirection of flow-retrograde as opposed to ante-grade- to the distal leg. This risk can be mitigated by placing a distal reperfusion cannula in another artery in the extremity to augment blood flow to the extremity. As with other peripheral vascular access, cannulation for VA ECMO can be additionally associated with the development of pseudoaneurysms and/or AV fistulization [2].

Hematologic Complications

Hematologic complications associated with ECMO are vast and can result in derangements of platelets, coagulation factors, and hemoglobin. Commonly cited complications that can be easily detected on screening serum diagnostics include hemolysis, hemodilution, and thrombocytopenia. As with other forms of extracorporeal support that are centered around the interaction of blood components with artificial surfaces and result in a degree of shear stress, ECMO therapy is no exception. These interactions can result in fibrin polymerization, platelet activation, release of microparticles, as well as result in the activation, functional alteration, and overall consumption of numerous coagulation factors [26]. It has been specifically associated with defects and consumption of multiple coagulation factors, fibrin formation, von Willebrand factor multimers, alterations in antithrombin levels, platelets, and fibrinogen [27]. Awareness of the potential for these complications, clinical monitoring for evidence of these and maintaining low threshold for obtaining additional diagnostics and/or replacement is crucial to management. As with other complications associated with this therapy, intrinsic pathology and the disease process that lead to initiation of ECMO support can also be contributory.

Gastrointestinal and Hepatobiliary Complications

As previously discussed injuries to vasculature and regional parenchyma can occur secondary to cannulation, this is not dissimilar in relation to risk of inferior vena cava and intrahepatic vasculature and/or hepatic parenchymal injury. Congestive hepatopathy with resultant impairment in hepatic function can additionally occur in the setting of venous congestion and/or inadequacy of drainage. Syndromes such as Budd-Chiari can develop in the setting of cannula misplacement and associated hepatic vein flow obstruction [28]. Impairments in flow and/or thromboembolic phenomena associated with VA ECMO can result in non-occlusive and/or acute focal mesenteric ischemia [29].

Renal or Genitourinary Complications

There are a few commonly encountered complications associated with either underlying disease pathology that prompted commencement of ECMO support (i.e., cardiogenic shock, acute tubular necrosis, and/or cardio-renal syndrome) or as a direct result of this therapy. Acute kidney injury is a prime example of this [30]. A commonly encountered etiology for acute kidney injury as a direct result of ECMO therapy is hemolysis and pigment-induced renal tubular injury. Management of this condition is centered around minimization of hemolysis, specifically ensuring adequacy of flow and oxygenator function, as well as minimization of pressure and turbulence. At times, renal replacement therapy utilization may be required [31]. Other complications that can be associated with this therapy in the setting of systemic anticoagulation include hematuria which can be similarly managed compared with those who suffer from this condition while not on ECMO support.

Emergencies and Catastrophic Events

While complications pose the most common risks to a patient on extracorporeal support, clinicians should also be aware of potential emergent and catastrophic events associated with this therapy. This section will focus on circuit air entrainment, accidental decannulation, pump failure, and pump head decoupling. When these situations occur, they must be addressed quickly or they can result in significant morbidity or even death of a patient.

Air

The entrainment of air into the extracorporeal circuit has been reported in approximately 4% of patients [32]. While uncommon, this complication can be catastrophic. Management of this complication is centered around ensuring that primary and secondary prevention strategies take place such as ensuring meticulous priming of the circuit, limiting access to the circuit, and utilizing tools such as ultrasonic bubble detectors and microfilters on intravenous sites [33].

Once air is detected, it requires rapid resolution from properly trained staff to prevent the pump ceasing to function due to being locked by the air and/or a potentially catastrophic air embolism from being transmitted to the patient. When air is identified in the circuit, one must take proper steps to ensure the air is not returned to the patient. The circuit should be clamped to trap air and prevent it from being transferred to the patient. The air should then be systematically manipulated back to the closest circuit outlet point for removal. If the air cannot be removed quickly utilizing this method (i.e., significant amount of air has been entrained), a circuit exchange must be expeditiously undertaken. For this reason, many centers keep a primed backup circuit available on units that care for ECLS patients [34].

Accidental Decannulation

Among the most fatal complications which can occur while a patient is on ECLS support is accidental decannulation happening in approximately 1.3% of patients, which is a true emergency as it can lead to mass air entrainment and catastrophic hemorrhage [32, 34, 35]. Many methods should be followed in order to prevent accidental decannulation. The most common causes of this emergency included improperly secured cannula, inadvertent removal of cannula dressing/sutures over time, or during migration and patient care (i.e., bathes, turning, or in transport) [36]. Each institution should have consistent processes for securing and suturing cannulas, as well as protocolized, regular assessment of cannula positioning to assess for migration. Confused or combative patients may require chemical or mechanical restraints. Should decannulation occur, the focus should be on ensuring existing cannula are clamped, ECMO support is ceased and attention is given to the primary vessel (i.e., holding pressure, performing primary vascular repair, transfusion, and resuscitation) until new access can be established and support can be resumed.

Pump Failure

With advances in technology, pump failure has drastically reduced. While extracorporeal pumps continue to pose risks, pump failure only occurs in 1.1% of patients [35]. Pump failure can be the result of a loss of power, or magnetic field imbalance in centrifugal pumps due to thrombosis, air, or pump head decoupling. The risk of pump failure due to power loss rarely occurs due to built-in backup batteries within many ECMO circuits. Most systems revert to battery power in the event of loss of electricity. Mechanical backups, such as hand cranking systems, also provide an additional method of prevention.

Magnetic field imbalance for centrifugal pumps is often mitigated with a secondary pump head being present at bedside (i.e., CentriMag system). In instances where thrombosis or air is the cause of this imbalance, these issues should be addressed as previously noted, or may require circuit exchange [37]. Pump decoupling, furthermore, may require complete reset of the system by turning off the console or turning the flow to zero. The pump may then need to be reset until the magnet and flow are resumed.

Conclusion

ECMO is an exceptionally complex, advanced form of extracorporeal life support that can be associated with various management complications and some may result in emergent situations (Fig. 8.4). There are several emergencies specific to ECMO therapy that all providers caring for patients on this support should not only be aware of, but prepared to manage. The best method of preventing complications and emergency situations is knowledge of the ECMO circuit and equipment being used, regional resources and backup resources, and protocols to include vigilant monitoring of patients who are receiving this therapy.

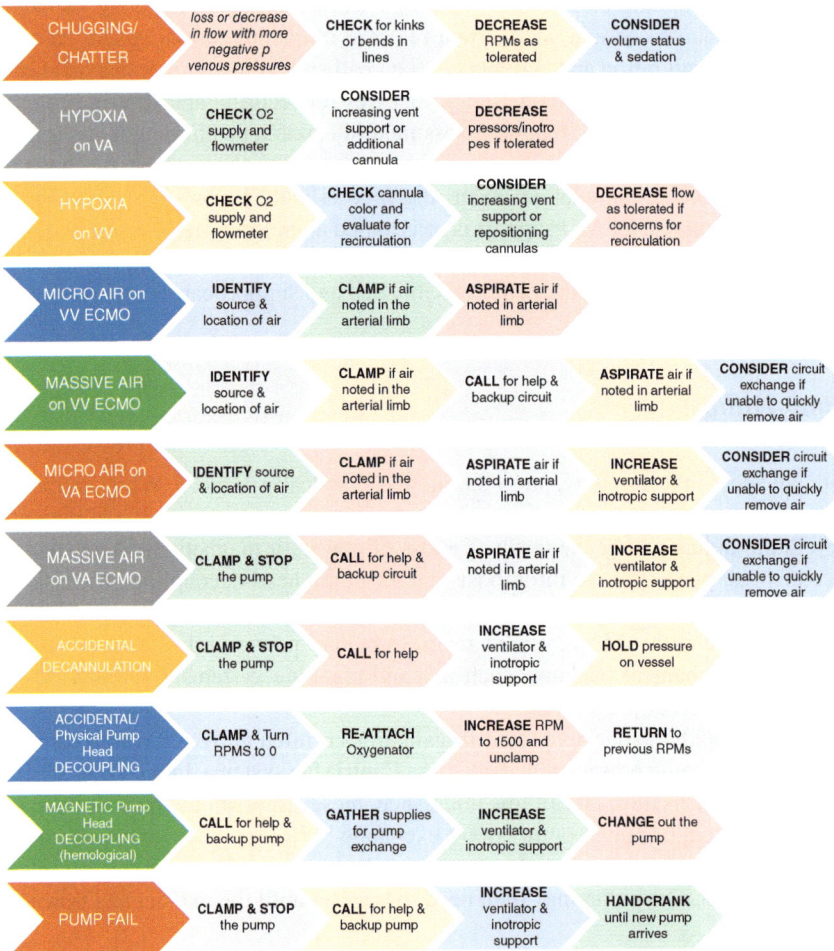

Fig. 8.4 Management of common complications and emergencies on ECMO

References

1. Zangrillo A, Landoni G, Biondi-Zoccai G, et al. A meta-analysis of complications and mortality of extracorporeal membrane oxygenation. Crit Care Resusc. 2013;15(3):172–8.
2. Pillai AK, Bhatti Z, Bosserman AJ, Mathew MC, Vaidehi K, Kalva SP. Management of vascular complications of extra-corporeal membrane oxygenation [Internet]. Cardiovasc Diagn Ther. 2018;8(3):372–7. Available from:. https://doi.org/10.21037/cdt.2018.01.11.
3. Sklar MC, Sy E, Lequier L, Fan E, Kanji HD. Anticoagulation practices during venovenous extracorporeal membrane oxygenation for respiratory failure. A systematic review. Ann Am Thorac Soc. 2016;13(12):2242–50.
4. Olson SR, Murphree CR, Zonies D, et al. Thrombosis and bleeding in extracorporeal membrane oxygenation (ECMO) without anticoagulation: a systematic review. ASAIO J. 2021;67(3):290–6.
5. Kurihara C, Walter JM, Karim A, et al. Feasibility of venovenous extracorporeal membrane oxygenation without systemic anticoagulation. Ann Thorac Surg. 2020;110(4):1209–15.
6. Wood KL, Ayers B, Gosev I, et al. Venoarterial-extracorporeal membrane oxygenation without routine systemic anticoagulation decreases adverse events [Internet]. Ann Thorac Surg. 2020;109(5):1458–66. Available from:. https://doi.org/10.1016/j.athoracsur.2019.08.040.
7. Makdisi G, Wang I-W. Extra corporeal membrane oxygenation (ECMO) review of a lifesaving technology. J Thorac Dis. 2015;7(7):E166–76.
8. Definition of THROMBOSIS [Internet]. [cited 2023 Jan 25]. Available from: https://www.merriam-webster.com/dictionary/thrombosis
9. Tang W, Zhang W-T, Zhang J, et al. Prevalence of hematologic complications on extracorporeal membranous oxygenation in critically ill pediatric patients: a systematic review and meta-analysis [Internet]. Thromb Res. 2023;222:75–84. Available from:. https://doi.org/10.1016/j.thromres.2022.12.014.
10. Ma M, Liang S, Zhu J, et al. The efficacy and safety of Bivalirudin versus heparin in the anti-coagulation therapy of extracorporeal membrane oxygenation: a systematic review and meta-analysis. Front Pharmacol. 2022;13:771563.
11. Biffi S, Di Bella S, Scaravilli V, et al. Infections during extracorporeal membrane oxygenation: epidemiology, risk factors, pathogenesis and prevention. Int J Antimicrob Agents. 2017;50(1):9–16.
12. Burket JS, Bartlett RH, Vander Hyde K, Chenoweth CE. Nosocomial infections in adult patients undergoing extracorporeal membrane oxygenation. Clin Infect Dis. 1999;28(4):828–33.
13. Mulla H. Drug disposition during extra-corporeal membrane oxygenation (Ecmo) [Internet]. Paediatr Clin Pharmacol. 2006:545–5. Available from: https://doi.org/10.1201/b14101-59.
14. Sutiman N, Koh JC, Watt K, et al. Pharmacokinetics alterations in critically ill pediatric patients on extracorporeal membrane oxygenation: a systematic review [Internet]. Available from: https://doi.org/10.21203/rs.2.19089/v1.
15. Walter JM, Kurihara C, Corbridge TC, Bharat A. Chugging in patients on veno-venous extracorporeal membrane oxygenation: an under-recognized driver of intravenous fluid administration in patients with acute respiratory distress syndrome? Heart Lung. 2018;47(4):398–400.
16. Website [Internet]. Available from: https://doi.org/10.1016/j.jtcvs.2016.10.067.
17. Boissier E, Lakhal K, Senage T, et al. Haemolysis index: validation for haemolysis detection during extracorporeal membrane oxygenation. Br J Anaesth. 2020;125(2):e218–20.
18. Omar HR, Mirsaeidi M, Socias S, et al. Plasma free hemoglobin is an independent predictor of mortality among patients on extracorporeal membrane oxygenation support. PLoS One. 2015;10(4):e0124034.
19. Tonna JE, Abrams D, Brodie D, et al. Management of adult patients supported with venovenous extracorporeal membrane oxygenation (VV ECMO): guideline from the extracorporeal life support organization (ELSO) [Internet]. ASAIO J. 2021;67(6):601–10. Available from:. https://doi.org/10.1097/mat.0000000000001432.

20. [No title] [Internet]. [cited 2023 Jan 25]. Available from: https://www.elso.org/portals/0/files/elso_recirculation_guideline_may2015.pdf
21. St-Arnaud C, Thériault M-M, Mayette M. North-south syndrome in veno-arterial extracorporeal membrane oxygenator: the other Harlequin syndrome [Internet]. Can J Anesth/J Can Anesth. 2020;67(2):262–3. Available from:. https://doi.org/10.1007/s12630-019-01501-w.
22. Wasyluk W, Zwolak A. Metabolic alterations in sepsis. J Clin Med Res [Internet]. 2021;10(11). Available from: https://doi.org/10.3390/jcm10112412.
23. Mehta A, Ibsen LM. Neurologic complications and neurodevelopmental outcome with extracorporeal life support. Pediatr Crit Care Med. 2013;2(4):40–7.
24. Roumy A, Liaudet L, Rusca M, Marcucci C, Kirsch M. Available from: pulmonary complications associated with veno-arterial extra-corporeal membrane oxygenation: a comprehensive review. Crit Care. 2020;24:212. https://doi.org/10.1186/s13054-020-02937-z.
25. Becker JA, Short BL, Martin GR. Cardiovascular complications adversely affect survival during extracorporeal membrane oxygenation. Crit Care Med. 1998;26(9):1582–6.
26. Granja T, Hohenstein K, Schüssel P, et al. Multi-modal characterization of the coagulopathy associated with extracorporeal membrane oxygenation. Crit Care Med. 2020;48(5):e400–8.
27. Website [Internet]. Available from: Cartwright B, Bruce HM, Kershaw G, et al. Hemostasis, coagulation and thrombin in venoarterial and venovenous extracorporeal membrane oxygenation: the HECTIC study. Sci Rep. 2021;11:7975. https://doi.org/10.1038/s41598-021-87026-z.
28. Victor K, Barrett N, Glover G, Kapetanakis S, Langrish C. Acute Budd–Chiari syndrome during veno-venous extracorporeal membrane oxygenation diagnosed using transthoracic echocardiography [Internet]. Br J Anaesth. 2012;108(6):1043–4. Available from:. https://doi.org/10.1093/bja/aes161.
29. Renaudier M, de Roux Q, Bougouin W, et al. Acute mesenteric ischaemia in refractory shock on veno-arterial extracorporeal membrane oxygenation [Internet]. Eur Heart J Acute Cardiovasc Care. 2021;10(1):62–70. Available from:. https://doi.org/10.1177/2048872620915655.
30. Ostermann M, Lumlertgul N. Acute kidney injury in ECMO patients. Crit Care. 2021;25(1):313.
31. Ostermann M, Connor M Jr, Kashani K. Continuous renal replacement therapy during extracorporeal membrane oxygenation: why, when and how? Curr Opin Crit Care. 2018;24(6):493–503.
32. Butt W, Heard M, Peek GJ. Clinical management of the extracorporeal membrane oxygenation circuit [Internet]. Pediatr Crit Care Med. 2013;14:S13–9. Available from:. https://doi.org/10.1097/pcc.0b013e318292ddc8.
33. Zanatta P, Forti A, Bosco E, et al. Microembolic signals and strategy to prevent gas embolism during extracorporeal membrane oxygenation. J Cardiothorac Surg. 2010;5:5.
34. Chan KM, Wan WTP, Ling L, So JMC, Wong CHL, Tam SBS. Management of circuit air in extracorporeal membrane oxygenation: a single center experience [Internet]. ASAIO J. 2022;68(3):e39–43. Available from:. https://doi.org/10.1097/mat.0000000000001494.
35. Kim DH, Cho WH, Son J, Lee SK, Yeo HJ. Catastrophic mechanical complications of extracorporeal membrane oxygenation. ASAIO J. 2021;67(9):1000–5.
36. Bull T, Corley A, Lye I, Spooner AJ, Fraser JF. Cannula and circuit management in peripheral extracorporeal membrane oxygenation: an international survey of 45 countries. PLoS One. 2019;14(12):e0227248.
37. Lubnow M, Philipp A, Foltan M, et al. Technical complications during veno-venous extracorporeal membrane oxygenation and their relevance predicting a system-exchange – retrospective analysis of 265 cases. PLoS One. 2014;9(12):e112316.

Chapter 9
Patient Care while on ECMO

Molly Johnson, Kyle Gronbeck, and Shaun L. Thompson

Objectives

1. Discuss practices for day-to-day care for patients on ECMO support
2. Review methods and practice of transport of patients on ECMO
3. Review hemodynamic monitoring interventions for ECMO patients
4. Discuss difficulties with sedation while on ECMO and use of paralytic agents
5. Overview of rehabilitation on ECMO and nutritional needs

Introduction

The use of extracorporeal membrane oxygenation (ECMO) continues to expand worldwide and is becoming a common method of support for critically ill patients in modern intensive care units. The day-to-day care of these patients can be extremely complex, and even simple care measures can be challenging due to the tenuous situation that these patients find themselves in when on ECMO support. From daily nursing cares, hemodynamic and neurologic monitoring, and transport of patients while on ECMO requires specialized training and understanding of how ECMO affects these practices. Inability to perform these maneuvers safely and appropriately can lead to potential morbidity and poor outcomes in this complex patient cohort.

M. Johnson · K. Gronbeck · S. L. Thompson (✉)
University of Nebraska Medical Center, Omaha, NE, USA
e-mail: slthomps@unmc.edu

Basic Care Considerations

Day-to-day care of ECMO patients requires specialized training for not only physicians, but also nursing staff and other providers such as clinical perfusionists and respiratory therapists. Monitoring of all aspects of ECMO circuit is performed on an hourly basis along with all other vital signs and clinical indicators for critically ill patients. Patients on ECMO require some specialized care considerations which will be discussed in this chapter.

Cannula Care and Monitoring

Patients on ECMO should receive standard critical care nursing. However, there are some specific assessments and cares required. These nursing cares and assessments are targeted to identify potential complications early. Safe cannula care and evaluation during ECMO are critical to prevent complications such as cannula-related infections, mechanical circuit dysfunction, cannula dislodgment which can lead to air embolism, hemorrhage, or loss of ECMO flow. These complications can be life threatening, and steps to reduce the risk should be implemented. Cannula site and depth should be assessed and documented at minimum every hour [1, 2]. Chlorhexidine gluconate (CHG) impregnated dressings should be used to cover the cannulation site unless contraindicated [1, 3]. Contraindications may include copious drainage, active bleeding, and allergy to CHG. The dressing should be changed at least every 7 days, and some centers change more frequently [1, 3]. The dressing should be changed immediately if dressing integrity is compromised, the line has potential to be exposed or if any of the following criteria are met: drainage outside CHG square, drainage >1 inch from insertion site for non-CHG dressings, and CHG square saturated when applicable [1]. The cannula and tubing may cause pressure injuries to the underlying skin. Frequent repositioning of the tubing and applying dressings as a barrier between the cannula and the skin may prevent further injury [2].

Securing the cannula is critical to prevent catastrophic complications such as cannula dislodgment, air entrainment, or bleeding. Bull et al. in a larger international survey suggested that one-third of respondents reported an incident of a cannula malposition, dislodgment, or accidental decannulation leading to an adverse patient outcome [3]. Most centers choose to suture the cannulas in place while others use suture-less securing devices (image 1) [3]. Regardless of method of securement, the cannula must be secured at multiple points. In awake patients that tend to bend their legs, you may consider placing a knee immobilizer to minimize the movement of the cannula and accidental dislodgment.

During peripheral veno-arterial ECMO, there is additional risk of distal limb ischemia from reduced blood flow and oxygen delivery to the lower extremity distal to the insertion point of the cannula. Recent studies suggest that incidence of limb ischemia ranges from 10% to 22% [4, 5]. The proposed mechanisms include suboptimal perfusion due to the underlying disease, peripheral vascular disease, dissection of the artery, thrombosis, distal emboli, and cannula size that nearly occludes the vessel [5, 6]. Distal perfusion cannulas are discussed in another chapter.

Near-infrared spectroscopy (NIRS) is a tool utilized to detect signs of poor tissue oxygenation. Unlike pulse oximetry, it monitors the difference between oxyhemoglobin and deoxyhemoglobin, and pulsatile blood flow is not required for an accurate reading. Studies have shown that a NIRS saturation of below 50% for more than four minutes correlates to limb ischemia with a positive predictive value of 86% [7]. Utilizing this technology should not replace frequent limb and vascular site assessments which should still be completed every hour [1, 2].

Nutrition for the ECMO Patient

Patients requiring ECMO support are usually the most severely ill patient in that intensive care unit. Because of the treatment that they are undergoing and the severity of their illness, ECMO patients are many times bed bound, immobile, and under deep sedation for many days at a time. As with any other critically ill patient in this situation, the need for adequate nutrition is paramount but the use of ECMO can pose challenges and risks to the use of enteral nutrition [8]. Risks of enteral nutrition in this patient population included intolerance of enteral feeding all the way to severe complications such as acute mesenteric ischemia [9]. Patients may require high dose vasopressor agents and concerns for decreased gastric motility have all been cited as reasons to withhold initiation of enteral feeding [8, 10]. Despite these risks, it has been shown that early enteral nutrition in this patient population can be safe to perform, but can also decrease in-hospital and 28 day mortality [8–10].

Determination of energy expenditure and amount of calories needed per day for critically ill patients is best determined using indirect calorimetry [10]. This can be a challenge for the patient on ECMO due to the presence of the membrane lung that artificially removes carbon dioxide. Since indirect calorimetry uses the amount of carbon dioxide produced to help and determine caloric needs, this can lead to confusion and difficulty in accurate calculations for this patient population [10]. The methods of measurement performed in studies to determine energy expenditure have not been validated and also require equipment that is not readily available at most centers [10, 11]. Because of this, caloric needs are typically estimation-based available guidelines for critically ill patients [10]. The range of kilocalories per kilogram varies from 20 to 30 kcal/kg depending upon the societal guidelines that are referenced, but most guidelines agree that 25 kcal/kg is a safe estimate of caloric needs for patients requiring ECMO support [10]. Once needs are determined, it has been shown to start enteral nutrition at a slow or trophic rate and incrementally increase [9]. This way, if the patient has intolerance to enteral nutrition or develops other complications such as intestinal ischemia, the nutrition can be stopped and other methods of feeding can be utilized such as parenteral nutrition.

Once caloric goals are known, the composition of enteral nutrition is something that needs to be determined. Different formulations of enteral nutrition exist, and some research has been done on these differing formulations for the critically ill patient. When it comes to the best formulation for patient requiring ECMO, there is no such data to strongly support the use of one version over the other [8, 10].

Depending on the formulation chosen, the amount of protein that patients receive on a daily basis is important to help lessen skeletal muscle loss that occurs not only for patients on ECMO support, but also for any critically ill patient [10, 12]. The limited data thus far has shown that providing patients on ECMO 1.2 g/kg/d of protein in their enteral nutrition should be sufficient for daily needs [10]. Attaining these goals has been shown to be reached in >80% of patients so providing this therapy is feasible for patients on ECMO [10, 13]. Again, a stepwise increase in the rate of enteral nutrition should be employed to avoid potential intolerance of feeding and to monitor for more feared complications of enteral nutrition such as mesenteric ischemia [9, 14–16].

If enteral nutrition cannot be safely administered, parenteral nutrition can be a safe alternative. It is much less commonly used for patients on ECMO, with reports of use in 4–30% of patients on ECMO [10]. If parenteral nutrition is chosen, careful monitoring of the ECMO circuit must be performed as infiltration of lipids can occur in the membrane lung [10, 17]. This accumulation can lead to failure of the membrane lung and potential decompensation of the patient. This complication can also be accelerated if other lipid-containing medications are used simultaneously [10]. Monitoring of triglyceride levels and switching to non-lipid containing parenteral nutrition may occur if triglyceride levels become elevated or if concerns arise that the ECMO circuit efficiency is being affected by components of the parenteral nutrition [10].

Hemodynamic Monitoring

Hemodynamic monitoring is used to assist in identifying abnormal physiology in critically ill patients [18]. The purpose of recognizing changes in hemodynamics is to intervene before further complications can arise [19]. Patients are placed on ECMO because conventional methods to address poor perfusion and refractory shock are unsuccessful [20]. The physiologic response to ECMO support is complex and changes depending on various clinical scenarios [21]. Adequate hemodynamic monitoring is important to the clinical care of patients requiring ECMO [22]. There are differences in the monitoring of patients between the two main ECMO modalities. From bedside examination to non-invasive and invasive measurement modalities, ECMO patients require frequent and consistent monitoring to assure optimal care and outcomes.

When assessing ECMO patients for tissue perfusion, it is important to note general exam findings indicative of poor perfusion. These findings include but are not limited to neurological status, skin temperature gradients, mottling, capillary refill, oliguria, and respiratory status [23–26]. Capillary refill and skin mottling have been shown to correlate with increasing morbidity and mortality, specifically in ECMO

[27]. Early identification and subsequent resuscitation will improve patient perfusion and outcomes. Physical exam alone, especially in patients on ECMO, will not identify inadequate perfusion and a proper resuscitation target alone [28, 29].

Pulse oximetry (SpO2) is vital for monitoring critically ill ICU patients. SpO2 is useful in monitoring of ECMO patients but is not without its limitations. Typically, SpO2 is considered accurate to within 2–3% of oxyhemoglobin SaO2 [30, 31]. In patients on ECMO, this range is 3–7.2% higher and more inaccurate [32]. This could be related to shear stress of the ECMO circuit leading to endogenous carbon monoxide build up from hemolysis in combination with less pulsatile flow [33–37]. Frequent SaO2 monitoring is recommended even with normal SpO2 readings [32]. Table 9.1 showcases typical monitoring modalities.

A minimum target goal SaO2 of 80% and PaO2 of >50 mmHg should be achieved for patients on ECMO [38]. Serial blood gases allow titration of the sweep gas to assist in proper management of the patients pCO2 and pH [39]. With frequent ABGs and SaO2 assessments, hypoxia can be differentiated in patients on ECMO. Some instances include Harlequin syndrome, north-south syndrome, or issues with the ECMO oxygenator [40].

Patients who are being managed on ECMO should have an arterial line for continuous waveform blood pressure monitoring and frequent ABG draws [26]. Ideally the arterial line should be placed in the right radial or brachial artery [41]. This is used to assess oxygenation of the right arm which will give an idea on the location of the "mixing cloud" of blood between the arterial cannula flow and native cardiac output [42]. If native cardiac output has recovered sufficiently, it may overcome ECMO flow. If pulmonary gas exchange is impaired, this would manifest as hypoxia in the arterial blood gas from the right arm and lead the clinician to either make ventilator changes or possibly increase ECMO flows to move the mixing cloud further up toward the right innominate artery.

Arterial pressure waveform on the arterial line can give insight into how the heart is functioning in patients on VA ECMO. Pulse pressure monitoring via pulsatility on the arterial waveform is an indication of LV contractility [22]. A narrower or even flattened pulse pressure can indicate a decrease in the amount of left ventricular stroke volume [26]. A wider pulse pressure though does not necessarily indicate that a heart has recovered LV function. Other characteristics need to be evaluated for including individual patients' physiology and the current state of the shock they are experiencing. Flattened pulse pressure can indicate a low flow state through the native heart and even to a point of venous stasis [43]. This could lead to unwanted thrombosis, and the left ventricular should be decompressed. This can be done medically, surgically, or with percutaneous devices such as an Impella (Medtronic, Minneapolis, MN) or intra-aortic balloon pump [44]. The goal is to remedy the low flow state of the heart.

Mixed venous oxygen saturation (SvO2) is the percent of oxygen that is bound to hemoglobin in blood that has returned to the right side of the heart [45]. This can be conceptualized as the amount of oxygen that was not used by the tissues [46]. Classically, SvO2 is drawn from the tip of a pulmonary artery catheter as this is the last point of oxygen uptake before entering the pulmonary capillary bed [47]. Central venous oxygen saturation (ScvO2) is a surrogate for SvO2 and drawn not from a PAC, but from a central line such as an internal jugular or subclavian catheter

Table 9.1 Typical hemodynamic monitoring modalities

Monitor	Measurement	Normal values	Evaluation	Other considerations
SpO2 monitor	Peripheral oxygen saturation	Minimum target 80%, Goal >88%	Detects early hypoxia, poor perfusion, and ECMO specific disease such as Harlequin syndrome, north south syndrome, and malfunctioning ECMO oxygenator	Typically, accurate within 2–3% of SaO2 but range on ECMO is 3–7.2% higher
Arterial line	Continuous waveform blood pressure monitoring and frequent ABG draws	– Goal MAP >65mmHg – Goal PP >25 mmHG	Evaluates for hypotension, cardiac pulsatility, hypoxia/hypercarbia (ABGs)	Should be placed in the right arm of all VA ECMO patients
PAC (Swan-Ganz)	Cardiac output, cardiac index, pulmonary artery pressures, wedge pressure, SvO2	Normal SvO2 60–80% – RAP 0–7 mmHg – PASP 15–25 mmHg – PCWP 4–12 mmHg – CI: 2.8–3.2 – CO 5–6 lpm	SvO2 indicates global tissue perfusion and oxygenation. PAC can help determine volume status, cardiac output, and real-time cardiac function	PAC readings are inaccurate due to redirection of pulmonary blood flow from VA ECMO flow
In-line ScvO2	ScvO2 is a surrogate for SvO2	Normal ScvO2 >70%	Evaluates for tissue hypoxia as a surrogate for SvO2, in-line monitoring provides continuous real-time perfusion assessment	Low ScvO2 levels correlate to increased mortality on VA ECMO. Numbers are confounded by recirculation in VV ECMO
NIRS	Noninvasive monitoring of regional oxygen saturation	Device dependent, typically >60% is normal	Cerebral and extremity oxygen saturation, sudden changes in one extremity or one side of the brain can indicate ischemia (stroke, arterial occlusion)	NIRS is affected by changes in MAP, pCO2, ECMO flow, SpO2, hematocrit, temperature, sedation, and activity
Lactate	Surrogate lab value for optimal oxygen delivery	<2.3 mmol/L is normal	Trending lactate monitors clearance and improved tissue perfusion, higher levels and poor lactate clearance lead to increased mortality	Exogenous catecholamines, hepatic dysfunction, sepsis, cardiac surgery impact lactate levels outside of tissue perfusion

[48]. These measurements help to determine if the cardiac output is meeting the tissue demands of the patient. A normal SvO2 is between 60% and 80%. In cases of VA ECMO, an SvO2 is a reasonable indicator of global tissue perfusion and oxygenation [49]. Low ScvO2 can be secondary to increased metabolic rate, sepsis, or worsening cardiogenic shock and can be remedied by increasing oxygen supply, ECMO flow, or increased MAP [26]. Low ScvO2 levels on the circuit have been shown to correlate with increased mortality in VA ECMO [50].

Most modern ECMO circuits have the capability to provide in-line ScvO2 measurements. Since ScvO2 is a surrogate to SvO2, this is a continually measured mixed venous oxygen saturation and real-time assessment of tissue perfusion. VV ECMO patients present a unique dilemma as recirculation of blood in the circuit can falsely elevate ScvO2 readings. In the same manner, true SvO2 measurement from a PAC is confounded by the highly oxygenated blood returning from the oxygenator. If the site of measurement is too close to the ECMO return cannula in VV ECMO, the ScvO2 will be falsely elevated.

Near-infrared spectroscopy (NIRS) monitoring is a non-invasive method of estimating regional oxygen saturation [51]. This type of monitoring system is used in ECMO patients to monitor cerebral oxygen saturation [52]. In patients with cerebral NIRS monitoring, a unilateral decreased in rSO2 can indicate possible neurologic insult such as ischemic stroke, hemorrhagic stroke, or brain death [53]. Unfortunately, cerebral NIRS can be affected by MAP, pCO2, ECMO blood flow, SpO2 measurements, hematocrit, body temperature, and level of sedation [22].

NIRS monitoring is also used in extremities to monitor tissue perfusion of the arms and legs [7]. A lower rStO2 in one leg, such as the leg with the femoral cannula, can indicate lower extremity ischemia [54]. This is a significant complication of ECMO cannulation, and if addressed early could lead to salvage of ischemic extremities. Mostly if not all patients on ECMO should receive cerebral and extremity NIRS monitoring to evaluate for early development of ischemia.

Lactate levels can be monitored in a serial fashion for patients on ECMO as this acts as a surrogate for optimal oxygen delivery. Once ECMO has been initiated, it is important to trend lactate levels, to ensure clearance and improved tissue perfusion with this therapy [55]. Evidence has shown that high lactate levels at the initiation of ECMO, and higher lactate levels refractory to ECMO flow, prognosticates worse outcomes [56, 57]. It is important to note that there are other causes of hyperlactatemia other than poor tissue perfusion, and these should be evaluated for in all cases. These situations can include exogenous catecholamines, impaired liver function, sepsis, and post cardiac surgery patients [58].

Mobilization and Rehabilitation

With improved ECMO systems and technology, the ability to mobilize patients on ECMO is possible [59]. Literature supporting the mobilization and physical therapy of ICU patients has led to improvements in early rehabilitation for critically ill patients requiring ECMO [60].

Patients on ECMO are some of the most ill and labile patients in the hospital. Due to their instability and invasive devices, many of these patients require prolonged periods of immobility [61]. Bed rest is required because one of the major barriers to rehabilitation and mobility is the concern for cannula dislodgement [62]. This long period of bed rest has led to profound ICU-related myopathy, delayed recovery, and weakness present for months to years post ECMO [63]. Early ICU rehabilitation has been shown to improve long-term functional outcomes, muscle strength, and mobility [64]. The majority of literature supporting mobilization on ECMO is for patients on VV ECMO, predominately single site cannulation, awaiting native lung recovery, or lung transplantation. However, there is a role as well for patients who are on VA ECMO [65]. Overall, studies have reported that physical therapy and rehab in ECMO patients are safe, feasible, and worth the risk of adverse events [66]. Overall strategies for physical therapy and occupational therapy in patents on ECMO improve functional outcomes, reduce ICU delirium, and shorten overall ICU length of stays [66].

Factors that may inhibit rehabilitation strategies include profound delirium, high oxygen requirements, high PEEP requirements (which limits disconnecting from the ventilator), high levels of inotropic support, morbid obesity, and limited staffing resources [62]. In these instances, awake and interactive rehabilitation is unsafe, and patients need more time to stabilize before initiation. ECMO patients who are awake and spontaneously breathing have advantages to recovery such as improved V/Q mismatch, increased comfort, improved patient communication, and reduced chance of ventilator associated pneumonia [67]. If there is difficulty in getting patients to an awake, spontaneous breathing state, tracheostomy may be of benefit. Tracheostomy is useful for times of high ventilatory support, while maintaining little to no sedation and improving delirium [68]. It is inevitable that most patients on ECMO will require mechanical ventilation at some point but leaning on the ECMO circuit and weaning them from the ventilator as soon as possible with or without tracheostomy can be beneficial. Patients on VA ECMO are great candidates for awake ECMO and rehab as many of these patients have persevered lung function and are awaiting more long-term mechanical circulatory support such as a ventricular assist device or transplant [69]. Awakening these patients and participation in therapy will allow a speedier time to VAD and definitive therapy such as transplant. Patients awake on ECMO have overall shorter post-operative mechanical ventilation, better tolerance of physical therapy, and reduced multi-organ failure with an increase in chance of definitive therapies [62].

Ambulation and Cannula Positioning

ECMO patients are usually cannulated in a femoral-femoral fashion. Other techniques include internal jugular-femoral configuration where the femoral cannula is the drainage cannula for VV ECMO. Both of these configuration lead to disadvantages as the groin cannulas are sutured in allowing gravity to pull them down increasing risk of accidental decannulation during therapy [62]. If patients are awake and not sedated, patient discomfort and movement can lead to cannula movement, mispositioning, or kinking of the tubing which could impact flows and lead to decompensation. Most VA ECMO is done with at least one femoral cannula, or a central cannula. While these patients can be awake, ambulation and rehab may be difficult. Some institutions which are comfortable with these patients may have protocols in place for the ambulation of a femoral cannulated patient [70].

The preferred approach for awake and ambulating VV ECMO patients is a double-lumen single site cannula in the right internal jugular vein [71]. Such cannulas require special expertise in placement and are done in the operating room with TEE guidance, deep sedation, and usually fluoroscopy. Examples of these VV ECMO cannulas are the Avalon, or added RVAD support such as the Protek-duo [72]. Cannula securement needs to resist malposition with head and body movement, ambulation, and physical therapy.

Ambulation remains the primary goal of physical therapy in awakened ECMO patients but is resource demanding. Bed-based physical activities may require only one staff member to be present, while activities at the bedside can require up to three members [66]. If patients ambulate this may take up to 5 members to perform, including physical therapy, perfusionist, respiratory therapy, bedside nurses, and technicians. The primary general therapy goal is maintenance of muscles that contribute to the upright position and work against gravity, such as axial and core muscles [61]. This improves neck stability, core muscle strength, and hip mobility. These are key muscles to maintaining everyday upright mobility and are also quickly lost in the prolonged supinated patient [73]. Major adverse events with ambulation include accidental decannulation, displacement of the femoral cannula, bleeding at the cannula site, fracture of a cannula, thromboembolic events, and rarely cardiac arrest [74]. Major factors leading to increased ambulation include single site cannulation and upper body cannulation, low levels of sedation, and ECMO specialized teams, which are all factors in awake ECMO [75]. Overall early ambulation improves functional capacity of ICU patients [66]. Ambulation of patients on ECMO is safe and prevents serious neuromuscular complications and is possible in patients with femoral vessel cannulation with limited adverse events in the literature [76].

In-bed physical therapy techniques are primarily focused on positioning. Proper positioning is key in reducing pressure sores in ICU patients, and frequent repositioning can help maintain muscle strength [77]. Kinetic exercises and the use of bed-based equipment can assist in patients who are unable to ambulate, but also supplement ambulating awake ECMO patients [62]. This may include in-bed cycle ergometers, in-bed leg press devices, weights for lifting, and physical therapist driven stretching and range of motion. Muscle strengthening exercises should focus on neck, trunk control, and muscles used in sitting up and walking [78]. Sitting in bed chair or moving to the chair is important and can reduce delirium and improve core muscle strength in patients on ECMO. This reduces complications of bed sores and ICU-based myopathy and improves pulmonary complications [74]. Overall good rehabilitation includes passive movements of upper and lower limbs, proper positioning including upright positioning at all times, muscle strengthening exercises, sitting up bed chair mode, or in bedside chair, assist to stand with and without support, with primary goal of ambulation.

The dose of rehabilitation varies and is institution dependent. Ambulation ranges from standing and walking to bed chair (5–10 feet), to up to 30–850 meters [75]. The median distances walked in awake ECMO patients are 200–300 feet [74, 79, 80]. Progressive exercise and bed-based exercise are typically 20–60 minutes per day [81–83]. Patients who ambulate will typically tolerate and have longer sessions of physical therapy. Standing and ambulating at bedside for at least 10 minutes are beneficial, especially in instances where mobilizing large teams to walk in the hall are not feasible [74, 84, 85]. Cycling should be instituted when able for a minimum of 10 minutes as tolerated and can be done at bedside. Some patients on single site VV ECMO may tolerate up to 30 minutes out of bed in a recumbent bike [73, 86, 87]. Institutional goals for therapy sessions should be 20–90-minute sessions daily in awake ECMO patients, multiple days per week. Therapy should be progressive in nature, institution dependent, and patient directed depending on their own progress, goals, and abilities. The intensity of the exercise should be suited to meet each individual patient's needs [74]. ECMO settings may need to be changed such as flow, sweep gas flow, or $FiO2$ of the circuit and adjusted to maintain $PaO2 > 60$, $SvO2$ at 50% and a normal lactic acid [88]. For less invasive monitoring, $SpO2$ should be titrated to >88% monitored during each session. Equipment to consider includes cycle ergometers such as in-bed and recumbent bikes, upright cycle, tilt table, gait aid/walking frames, treadmill, rehabilitation chairs for passive transfer, hand weights, resistance bands, and in-bed leg press devices. Staff needs include physical therapists, occupational therapists, nursing staff, nursing technicians, perfusionists, and physicians [74]. With a multidisciplinary team and institutional protocols, regular physical therapy sessions are possible and recommended for all patients who require ECMO for a prolonged period of time.

Transport of the ECMO Patient

Patients on ECMO will frequently require transport of some form during their time on ECMO. This transport may be within the hospital for diagnostic or therapeutic studies and interventions. It may also require transport to another hospital system for ECMO services or specialized care such as heart or lung transplant [2].

Intra-Hospital Transport

Transport within the hospital is commonly required when ECMO patients require diagnostic or therapeutic interventions (CT imaging, IR, cath lab, OR). Even short transports within a hospital require preparation, coordination and have some risk of

Blood flow low limit alarm (mL/min)	
Blood flow high limit alarm (mL/min)	
Oxygen connectors secure	
Tubing clamps	
Cerebral saturation monitoring	
Backup console/ hand crank	
Total circuit inspection	
Oxygen tank	

Fig. 9.1 Example of intrahospital transport ECMO safety checklist courtesy of University of Nebraska Medical Center

complication due to the high acuity of the patient and the number of devices that are mobilized with the patient. These diagnostic or therapeutic interventions yield crucial information that often changes management [89]. Therefore, that risk must be weighed against the benefit from the proposed intervention. This patient movement should involve a team approach, and the healthcare team members may vary depending on the ECMO center. The teams often include an ECMO specialist, perfusionist, and the bedside nurse. We recommend completing a full safety checklist before and after transportation, see Fig. 9.1. This includes but is not limited to reviewing and documenting blood flow in low and high limit alarm settings, checking the oxygen connectors are secure, evaluating for chatter in the lines, ensuring tubing clamps are available, functional cerebral saturation monitoring, locate the backup console and hand crank are available, inspect the entire circuit including cannula sites, verify there is an oxygen tank available [1]. Non-circuit related checks should also include ventilator assessment or switching to transport ventilator and ensure adequate amounts of continuous infusions are available for the transport.

Inter-Hospital Transport

Inter-hospital transport of patients on ECMO is required when the referring facility does not have ECMO capabilities or a patient on ECMO requires specialized definitive management such as heart or lung transplant. The first documented inter-hospital ECMO transport was by Bartlett et al. in 1975 since that time inter-hospital transport has increased in frequency. This is multifactorial and related to the overall increase in ECMO utilization. Transport to high volume ECMO centers has been shown to reduce mortality [90]. The International ECMO Network suggests a "hub and spoke" model to safely deploy this resource to referring hospitals with no ECMO capabilities or limited ECMO capabilities [91]. This model allows consolidating ECMO care to high volume centers. Most of the internationally experienced centers providing ECMO transport utilize this "hub and spoke" model to regionalize ECMO [92].

These transports can be defined as primary or secondary. Primary is one where the receiving ECMO center sends a team to perform cannulation at the referring hospital prior and then transports the patient on ECMO. This may also occur when the referring hospital has the capability to cannulate for ECMO but not the resources to maintain ECMO support. In this case, the referring team does the cannulation to stabilize the patient and then the transport process is initiated immediately after. Secondary transport occurs when the patient is already on ECMO but is transferred to another facility for reasons other than ECMO support such as transplant consideration or durable mechanical circulatory support [92]. Indications for transport vary depending on the referral and receiving centers. In general, patients with reversible respiratory or cardiac failure that have an unacceptable risk of deteriorating en route should be considered candidates [93, 94]. A multidisciplinary conference call between hospitals is recommended prior to initiating ECMO and transportation. Involved team members should include cannulating surgeon, ECMO intensivist, ICU charge nurse, ECMO specialist, transport coordinator, other involved teams at receiving hospital (heart failure, interventional cardiology, lung transplant, etc.), as well as the referring hospital team (intensivist, cardiology, cardiac surgery, etc.).

Sedation and Paralysis Considerations

There are factors that impact the pharmacokinetics and pharmacodynamics of drugs in relation to patients in critical illness [95]. Patient specific factors include serum protein, acid-base imbalances, end organ abnormalities, and physiologic changes in sepsis [96]. Drug factors include lipophilicity, molecular size, and protein binding [97]. There are special factors in ECMO that impact PK and PD including the membrane oxygenator, circuit tubing, large bore cannulas, and fluid priming [98]. Lipophilicity is the octanol/water partition coefficient (abbreviated Log P) and is defined as the ratio of a drugs concentration that is soluble in the octanol phase to the concentration soluble in the aqueous phase [99]. Higher positive values indicate increased lipophilicity. This will be an important concept moving forward as lipophilic drugs have a high likelihood of sequestration due to solubility in the ECMO circuit [100]. Over time, protein deposits along the walls of ECMO tubing. This can lead to highly protein bound drugs binding to that protein, and in turn binding into the circuit [95]. Highly protein bound drugs will have a higher likelihood of sequestration over time.

When looking at different types of drug factors, hydrophilic agents tend to have a lower volume of distribution with low Log P values [101]. Overall critical illness and ECMO increase the volume of distribution of these agents. Contrast to lipophilic agents who have a high volume of distribution and Log P, where in critical illness and ECMO, there is a theoretical increase in volume of distribution and clearance [100]. Thus, renally cleared medications typically are not impacted by ECMO (hydrophilic) and hepatically cleared medications see an increased clearance (lipophilic), see Table 9.2.

Table 9.2 Pharmacokinetic and pharmacodynamic properties of commonly used sedatives, analgesics, and paralytic agents

Drug	LogP	Protein binding	Volume of distribution in ECMO	Sequestration (severe, moderate, mild)	Hydrophilic or lipophilic	Circuit extraction	Other considerations
Opioids							
Fentanyl	4.05	79–87%	Increased	Severe	Lipophilic	Ex vivo: 3% recovered at 24 hours, Trials: Twice the MME required compared to HM	May be useful for circumstances where short-term analgesia and sedation is required (procedures) Most sequestration of all the three main opioids
Hydromorphone	0.9	8–19%	Likely moderate increase	Mild	Hydrophilic	Ex vivo: 23% decrease at 12 hours compared to 55% with fentanyl. Trials: Required half MME compared to fentanyl, less time requiring deep sedation. Less delirium compared to fentanyl	Preferred agent, long half-life can be used in bolus or continuous dosing. Likely the lease circuit sequestration or comparable to morphine
Morphine	0.89	20–35%	Moderate increase	Mld to moderate	Hydrophilic	Ex vivo: 97% recovered at 24 hours In vivo:	Histamine release and accumulation of active metabolites in renal failure limit use
Sedatives							
Propofol	3.79	95–99%	Increased	Severe	Significantly lipophilic	Ex vivo: negligible amounts recovered at 24 hours In vitro: 70–75% lost at 120 minutes	Cardio-suppressive and causes hypotension. Highly lipophilic and protein bound. Mainly used for procedures and short-term sedation needs
Midazolam	3.89	97%	Increased	Severe	Significantly lipophilic	Ex vivo: 11–13% recovered at 24 hours	Active metabolites accumulate over time, exacerbated by liver and renal failure

(continued)

Table 9.2 (continued)

Drug	LogP	Protein binding	Volume of distribution in ECMO	Sequestration (severe, moderate, mild)	Hydrophilic or lipophilic	Circuit extraction	Other considerations
Dexmedetomidine	3.39	94%	Increased	Severe	Significantly lipophilic	In vitro: 76–89% lost by 24 hours	Patients able to be awake and interactive. Less useful if patient requiring deep sedation or is bradycardic
Ketamine	2.9	47%	Unknown	Unknown	Lipophilic	Studies: Decrease in vasopressor requirements and a decrease in sedation requirements	Can cause tachycardia and may impact patients with coronary artery disease negatively
Paralytics							
Cisatracurium	−3.73 (Log D)	38%	Unknown	Unknown	Less lipophilic	N/A	Low lipophilicity, Hoffman elimination and not affected by renal or hepatic systems Likely lowest ECMO sequestration compared to the other common agents
Rocuronium	−1.68 (Log D)	46%	Unknown	Unknown	More lipophilic	N/A	Primary hepatic elimination with some renal. Less lipophilic than vecuronium
Vecuronium	−0.75 (Log D)	70%	Unknown	Unknown	More lipophilic	N/A	Primary hepatic elimination with some renal

The main ECMO circuit factors that impact the pharmacokinetics of drugs in ECMO are fluid priming, augmented cardiac output, the membrane oxygenator, and circuit tubing [95]. Priming of the ECMO circuit with crystalloid when initiating ECMO can lead to hemodilution increasing the volume of distribution of drugs [102, 103]. Cardiac support from the ECMO pump increases blood flow through organs including the kidneys and liver, which increases drug metabolism and clearance. Lastly, drug sequestration plays a large role in patients on ECMO. Drugs are sequestered within the ECMO circuit due to lipophilicity and protein binding described above. The primary component of the ECMO circuit that leads to sequestration is the circuit tubing and membrane oxygenator [104]. The circuit components are composed of polyvinyl chloride (PVC), polymethylpentene, and silicone rubber, which are organic materials in which lipophilic medications can be absorbed and lead to increased volume of distribution [105].

Current ELSO guidelines recommend thorough sedation during ECMO cannulation and management for the first 12–24 hours [2]. This is to avoid complications such as spontaneous breathing, which may cause an embolism during cannulation. Movement of the patient can also make cannulations more difficult and longer, leading to increased complications with the procedure itself. After the first 12 to 24 hours post cannulation, sedation should be minimal and held in regular intervals. There is no specific guideline on medication selection and/or dosing regimen for patients on ECMO.

The sedative agents most commonly used in ECMO are propofol, dexmedetomidine, and midazolam [106]. The analgesic agents most commonly used are fentanyl, morphine, and hydromorphone [107]. Most sedative agents have a high percentage of protein binding and Log P, indicating lipophilicity and high sequestration in the ECMO circuit. In contrast, the analgesics behave differently from one another [101]. Fentanyl has higher protein binding and Log P values, meaning high doses are needed to achieve affect due to lipophilicity and circuit binding [101, 108]. Morphine and hydromorphone are sequestered less, with hydromorphone being considered the least protein bound [101, 109, 110]. For this reason, opioids have become a mainstay in the sedation and analgesia for patients on ECMO.

Paralysis Considerations

Neuromuscular blockade in ARDS is typically used to prevent ventilator asynchrony and to help improve oxygenation by attempting to increase compliance [111]. When patients have been initiated onto VV ECMO for ARDS, it is because conventional methods have failed [112]. To assist in the recovery process and rest the lungs, neuromuscular blockade is sometimes used during ECMO [113]. Unfortunately, there are adverse events with neuromuscular blockade including impaired diaphragmatic function and critical illness-related myopathy [114]. Neuromuscular agents have similarly impaired usage in ECMO to sedatives and opioids, with circuit sequestration and increasing doses being required to achieve proper neuromuscular blockade [115]. Cisatracurium is typically the preferred neuromuscular blocking agent in ECMO. This is primarily due to lower lipophilicity, more rapid onset, and not being impacted by hepatic or renal failure in metabolism and elimination [116]. Cisatracurium undergoes Hoffman elimination and does not rely on the hepatic or renal system for metabolism [117]. With lower lipophilicity, cisatracurium is bound in the ECMO circuit less than other agents. Vecuronium and rocuronium are more lipophilic and undergo hepatic and renal elimination pathways [118]. ECMO patients are critically ill and many suffer from renal and hepatic failure, making it problematic for medications that rely on these pathways [119, 120]. If cisatracurium is unavailable, frequent boluses of rocuronium and vecuronium in addition to higher rate of infusions may be needed but will likely also be effective.

References

1. Scriven N, PK, Knott J. UNMC ECMO nursing care protocols. 2022.
2. Brogan TV, LL, Lorusso R, MacLaren G, Peek G. Extracorporeal life support: the ELSO red book, vol 5, p 832; 2017.
3. Bull T, et al. Cannula and circuit management in peripheral extracorporeal membrane oxygenation: an international survey of 45 countries. PLoS One. 2019;14(12):e0227248.
4. Yang F, et al. Vascular complications in adult postcardiotomy cardiogenic shock patients receiving venoarterial extracorporeal membrane oxygenation. Ann Intensive Care. 2018;8(1):72.
5. Yau P, et al. Factors associated with ipsilateral limb ischemia in patients undergoing femoral cannulation extracorporeal membrane oxygenation. Ann Vasc Surg. 2019;54:60–5.
6. Bonicolini E, et al. Limb ischemia in peripheral veno-arterial extracorporeal membrane oxygenation: a narrative review of incidence, prevention, monitoring, and treatment. Crit Care. 2019;23(1):266.
7. Patton-Rivera K, Beck J, Fung K. Using near-infrared reflectance spectroscopy to assess distal-limb perfusion on venoarterial extracorporeal membrane oxygenation patients with femoral cannulation. Perfusion. 2018;33(8):618–23.
8. Davis RC 2nd, et al. Safety, tolerability, and outcomes of enteral nutrition in extracorporeal membrane oxygenation. Nutr Clin Pract. 2021;36(1):98–104.
9. Al-Dorzi HM, Arabi YM. Enteral nutrition safety with advanced treatments: extracorporeal membrane oxygenation, prone positioning, and infusion of neuromuscular blockers. Nutr Clin Pract. 2021;36(1):88–97.
10. Bear DE, Smith E, Barrett NA. Nutrition support in adult patients receiving extracorporeal membrane oxygenation. Nutr Clin Pract. 2018;33(6):738–46.
11. De Waele E, et al. Measuring resting energy expenditure during extracorporeal membrane oxygenation: preliminary clinical experience with a proposed theoretical model. Acta Anaesthesiol Scand. 2015;59(10):1296–302.
12. Hayes K, et al. Acute skeletal muscle wasting and relation to physical function in patients requiring extracorporeal membrane oxygenation (ECMO). J Crit Care. 2018;48:1–8.
13. MacGowan L, et al. Adequacy of nutrition support during extracorporeal membrane oxygenation. Clin Nutr. 2019;38(1):324–31.
14. Arabi YM, et al. Permissive underfeeding or standard enteral feeding in high- and low-nutritional-risk critically ill adults. Post Hoc analysis of the PermiT trial. Am J Respir Crit Care Med. 2017;195(5):652–62.

15. National Heart L, et al. Initial trophic vs full enteral feeding in patients with acute lung injury: the EDEN randomized trial. JAMA. 2012;307(8):795–803.
16. Taylor BE, et al. Guidelines for the provision and assessment of nutrition support therapy in the adult critically ill patient: Society of Critical Care Medicine (SCCM) and American Society for Parenteral and Enteral Nutrition (A.S.P.E.N.). Crit Care Med. 2016;44(2):390–438.
17. Buck ML, Ksenich RA, Wooldridge P. Effect of infusing fat emulsion into extracorporeal membrane oxygenation circuits. Pharmacotherapy. 1997;17(6):1292–5.
18. Boldt J. Clinical review: hemodynamic monitoring in the intensive care unit. Crit Care. 2002;6(1):52–9.
19. Antonelli M, et al. Hemodynamic monitoring in shock and implications for management. International consensus conference, Paris, France, 27–28 April 2006. Intensive Care Med. 2007;33(4):575–90.
20. Marasco SF, et al. Review of ECMO (extra corporeal membrane oxygenation) support in critically ill adult patients. Heart Lung Circ. 2008;17(Suppl 4):S41–7.
21. Ficial B, et al. Physiological basis of extracorporeal membrane oxygenation and extracorporeal carbon dioxide removal in respiratory failure. Membranes (Basel). 2021;11(3):225.
22. Krishnan S, Schmidt GA. Hemodynamic monitoring in the extracorporeal membrane oxygenation patient. Curr Opin Crit Care. 2019;25(3):285–91.
23. Ait-Oufella H, et al. Capillary refill time exploration during septic shock. Intensive Care Med. 2014;40(7):958–64.
24. Ait-Oufella H, et al. Mottling score predicts survival in septic shock. Intensive Care Med. 2011;37(5):801–7.
25. Brunauer A, et al. Changes in peripheral perfusion relate to visceral organ perfusion in early septic shock: a pilot study. J Crit Care. 2016;35:105–9.
26. Su Y, et al. Hemodynamic monitoring in patients with venoarterial extracorporeal membrane oxygenation. Ann Transl Med. 2020;8(12):792.
27. Zampieri FG, et al. Effects of a resuscitation strategy targeting peripheral perfusion status versus serum lactate levels among patients with septic shock. A Bayesian reanalysis of the ANDROMEDA-SHOCK trial. Am J Respir Crit Care Med. 2020;201(4):423–9.
28. Boerma EC, et al. Disparity between skin perfusion and sublingual microcirculatory alterations in severe sepsis and septic shock: a prospective observational study. Intensive Care Med. 2008;34(7):1294–8.
29. Hernandez G, et al. Effect of a resuscitation strategy targeting peripheral perfusion status vs serum lactate levels on 28 day mortality among patients with septic shock: the ANDROMEDA-SHOCK randomized clinical trial. JAMA. 2019;321(7):654–64.
30. Nitzan M, Romem A, Koppel R. Pulse oximetry: fundamentals and technology update. Med Devices (Auckl). 2014;7:231–9.
31. Perkins GD, et al. Do changes in pulse oximeter oxygen saturation predict equivalent changes in arterial oxygen saturation? Crit Care. 2003;7(4):R67.
32. Nisar S, et al. Pulse oximetry is unreliable in patients on veno-venous extracorporeal membrane oxygenation caused by unrecognized carboxyhemoglobinemia. ASAIO J. 2020;66(10):1105–9.
33. Brodie D, Bacchetta M. Extracorporeal membrane oxygenation for ARDS in adults. N Engl J Med. 2011;365(20):1905–14.
34. Kai Man C, Koon Ngai L. Endogenous carbon monoxide production in extracorporeal membrane oxygenation-related hemolysis: potential use of point-of-care CO-oximetry carboxyhemoglobin to detect hemolysis. Clin Case Rep. 2018;6(2):346–9.
35. Severinghaus JW, Spellman MJ Jr. Pulse oximeter failure thresholds in hypotension and vasoconstriction. Anesthesiology. 1990;73(3):532–7.
36. Subramanian VA, Berger RL. Carbon monoxide accumulation during extracoporeal membrane oxygenation for acute respiratory failure. Ann Thorac Surg. 1976;22(2):195–8.
37. Tripathi RS, Papadimos TJ. ECMO and endogenous carboxyhemoglobin formation. Int J Crit Illn Inj Sci. 2011;1(2):168.

38. Bartlett RH. Physiology of gas exchange during ECMO for respiratory failure. J Intensive Care Med. 2017;32(4):243–8.
39. Strassmann S, et al. Impact of sweep gas flow on extracorporeal CO2 removal (ECCO2R). Intensive Care Med Exp. 2019;7(1):17.
40. Patel B, Arcaro M, Chatterjee S. Bedside troubleshooting during venovenous extracorporeal membrane oxygenation (ECMO). J Thorac Dis. 2019;11(Suppl 14):S1698–707.
41. Rao P, et al. Venoarterial extracorporeal membrane oxygenation for cardiogenic shock and cardiac arrest. Circ Heart Fail. 2018;11(9):e004905.
42. Mossadegh C. Monitoring the ECMO. In: Mossadegh C, Combes A, editors. Nursing care and ECMO. Cham: Springer International Publishing; 2017. p. 45–70.
43. Hofer A, et al. Differential diagnosis of alterations in arterial flow and tissue oxygenation on venoarterial extracorporeal membrane oxygenation. Int J Artif Organs. 2017;40(11):651–5.
44. Cevasco M, et al. Left ventricular distension and venting strategies for patients on venoarterial extracorporeal membrane oxygenation. J Thorac Dis. 2019;11(4):1676–83.
45. Jain A, et al. Relation between mixed venous oxygen saturation and cardiac index. Nonlinearity and normalization for oxygen uptake and hemoglobin. Chest. 1991;99(6):1403–9.
46. Schumacker PT, Cain SM. The concept of a critical oxygen delivery. Intensive Care Med. 1987;13(4):223–9.
47. Squara P. Central venous oxygenation: when physiology explains apparent discrepancies. Crit Care. 2014;18(6):579.
48. Joshi R, de Witt B, Mosier JM. Optimizing oxygen delivery in the critically ill: the utility of lactate and central venous oxygen saturation (ScvO2) as a roadmap of resuscitation in shock. J Emerg Med. 2014;47(4):493–500.
49. Wagner K, et al. Is it possible to predict outcome in cardiac ECMO? Analysis of preoperative risk factors. Perfusion. 2007;22(4):225–9.
50. Han L, et al. Risk factors for refractory septic shock treated with VA ECMO. Ann Transl Med. 2019;7(18):476.
51. Taillefer MC, Denault AY. Cerebral near-infrared spectroscopy in adult heart surgery: systematic review of its clinical efficacy. Can J Anaesth. 2005;52(1):79–87.
52. Maldonado Y, Singh S, Taylor MA. Cerebral near-infrared spectroscopy in perioperative management of left ventricular assist device and extracorporeal membrane oxygenation patients. Curr Opin Anaesthesiol. 2014;27(1):81–8.
53. Pozzebon S, et al. Cerebral near-infrared spectroscopy in adult patients undergoing venoarterial extracorporeal membrane oxygenation. Neurocrit Care. 2018;29(1):94–104.
54. Kim DJ, et al. Near-infrared spectroscopy monitoring for early detection of limb ischemia in patients on veno-arterial extracorporeal membrane oxygenation. ASAIO J. 2017;63(5):613–7.
55. Li JW, et al. Change of lactic acid concentration in patients receiving extracorporeal membrane oxygenation. J Clin Rehab Tissue Eng Res. 2008;12:2789–92.
56. Merkle-Storms J, et al. Impact of lactate clearance on early outcomes in pediatric ECMO patients. Medicina (Kaunas). 2021;57(3):284.
57. Slottosch I, et al. Lactate and lactate clearance as valuable tool to evaluate ECMO therapy in cardiogenic shock. J Crit Care. 2017;42:35–41.
58. Andersen LW, et al. Etiology and therapeutic approach to elevated lactate levels. Mayo Clin Proc. 2013;88(10):1127–40.
59. Pacheco LD, Saade GR, Hankins GDV. Extracorporeal membrane oxygenation (ECMO) during pregnancy and postpartum. Semin Perinatol. 2018;42(1):21–5.
60. Ko Y, et al. Feasibility and safety of early physical therapy and active mobilization for patients on extracorporeal membrane oxygenation. ASAIO J. 2015;61(5):564–8.
61. Polastri M, et al. Physiotherapy for patients on awake extracorporeal membrane oxygenation: a systematic review. Physiother Res Int. 2016;21(4):203–9.
62. Haji JY, Mehra S, Doraiswamy P. Awake ECMO and mobilizing patients on ECMO. Indian J Thorac Cardiovasc Surg. 2021;37(Suppl 2):309–18.

63. Chen X, et al. Intensive care unit-acquired weakness in patients with extracorporeal membrane oxygenation support: frequency and clinical characteristics. Front Med (Lausanne). 2022;9:792201.
64. Iwai K, et al. Effect of early rehabilitation in the intensive care unit by a dedicated therapist using a rehabilitation protocol: a single-center retrospective study. Prog Rehabil Med. 2021;6:20210030.
65. Rehder KJ, et al. Active rehabilitation during extracorporeal membrane oxygenation as a bridge to lung transplantation. Respir Care. 2013;58(8):1291–8.
66. Ferreira DDC, et al. Safety and potential benefits of physical therapy in adult patients on extracorporeal membrane oxygenation support: a systematic review. Rev Bras Ter Intensiva. 2019;31(2):227–39.
67. Xia J, et al. Spontaneous breathing in patients with severe acute respiratory distress syndrome receiving prolonged extracorporeal membrane oxygenation. BMC Pulm Med. 2019;19(1):237.
68. Swol J, Strauch JT, Schildhauer TA. Tracheostomy as a bridge to spontaneous breathing and awake-ECMO in non-transplant surgical patients: tracheostomy as a bridge to spontaneous breathing and awake-ECMO. Eur J Heart Fail. 2017;19:120–3.
69. Abrams D, Garan AR, Brodie D. Awake and fully mobile patients on cardiac extracorporeal life support. Ann Cardiothorac Surg. 2019;8(1):44–53.
70. Keshavamurthy S, et al. Ambulatory extracorporeal membrane oxygenation (ECMO) as a bridge to lung transplantation. Indian J Thorac Cardiovasc Surg. 2021;37(Suppl 3):366–79.
71. Bazan VM, et al. Overview of the bicaval dual lumen cannula. Indian J Thorac Cardiovasc Surg. 2021;37(Suppl 2):232–40.
72. Ngai C-W, Ng PY, Sin W-C. Bicaval dual lumen cannula in adult veno-venous extracorporeal membrane oxygenation—clinical pearls for safe cannulation. J Thorac Dis. 2018;10:S624–8.
73. Rahimi RA, et al. Physical rehabilitation of patients in the intensive care unit requiring extracorporeal membrane oxygenation: a small case series. Phys Ther. 2013;93(2):248–55.
74. Hayes K, et al. Rehabilitation of adult patients on extracorporeal membrane oxygenation: a scoping review. Aust Crit Care. 2022;35(5):575–82.
75. Abrams D, et al. Early mobilization during extracorporeal membrane oxygenation for cardiopulmonary failure in adults: factors associated with intensity of treatment. Ann Am Thorac Soc. 2022;19(1):90–8.
76. Pasrija C, et al. Ambulation with femoral arterial cannulation can be safely performed on venoarterial extracorporeal membrane oxygenation. Ann Thorac Surg. 2019;107(5):1389–94.
77. Hodgin KE, et al. Physical therapy utilization in intensive care units: results from a national survey. Crit Care Med. 2009;37(2):561–6; quiz 566–8.
78. Kourek C, et al. Modalities of exercise training in patients with extracorporeal membrane oxygenation support. J Cardiovasc Dev Dis. 2022;9(2):34.
79. Boling B, et al. Safety of nurse-led ambulation for patients on venovenous extracorporeal membrane oxygenation. Prog Transplant. 2016;26(2):112–6.
80. Hoopes CW, et al. Extracorporeal membrane oxygenation as a bridge to pulmonary transplantation. J Thorac Cardiovasc Surg. 2013;145(3):862–7; discussion 867–8.
81. Buchtele N, et al. Successful weaning from 65-day extracorporeal membrane oxygenation therapy in influenza-associated acute respiratory distress syndrome. Int J Artif Organs. 2016;39(5):249–52.
82. Liu K, et al. A progressive early mobilization program is significantly associated with clinical and economic improvement: a single-center quality comparison study. Crit Care Med. 2019;47(9):e744–52.
83. Mark A, et al. Maintaining mobility in a patient who is pregnant and has COVID-19 requiring extracorporeal membrane oxygenation: a case report. Phys Ther. 2021;101(1):pzaa189.
84. Chavez J, et al. Promotion of progressive mobility activities with ventricular assist and extracorporeal membrane oxygenation devices in a cardiothoracic intensive care unit. Dimens Crit Care Nurs. 2015;34(6):348–55.

85. Liu K, et al. The safety of a novel early mobilization protocol conducted by ICU physicians: a prospective observational study. J Intensive Care. 2018;6:10.
86. Blum JM, et al. Perioperative management of bridge-to-lung transplant using ECMO. ASAIO J. 2013;59(3):331–5.
87. Javidfar J, Bacchetta M. Bridge to lung transplantation with extracorporeal membrane oxygenation support. Curr Opin Organ Transplant. 2012;17(5):496–502.
88. Camboni D, et al. Possibilities and limitations of a miniaturized long-term extracorporeal life support system as bridge to transplantation in a case with biventricular heart failure. Interact Cardiovasc Thorac Surg. 2009;8(1):168–70.
89. Prodhan P, et al. Intrahospital transport of children on extracorporeal membrane oxygenation: indications, process, interventions, and effectiveness. Pediatr Crit Care Med. 2010;11(2):227–33.
90. Peek GJ, et al. Efficacy and economic assessment of conventional ventilatory support versus extracorporeal membrane oxygenation for severe adult respiratory failure (CESAR): a multicentre randomised controlled trial. Lancet. 2009;374(9698):1351–63.
91. Combes A, et al. Position paper for the organization of extracorporeal membrane oxygenation programs for acute respiratory failure in adult patients. Am J Respir Crit Care Med. 2014;190(5):488–96.
92. Broman LM, et al. International survey on extracorporeal membrane oxygenation transport. ASAIO J. 2020;66(2):214–25.
93. Labib A, et al. Extracorporeal life support organization guideline for transport and retrieval of adult and pediatric patients with ECMO support. ASAIO J. 2022;68(4):447–55.
94. Tipograf Y, et al. A decade of interfacility extracorporeal membrane oxygenation transport. J Thorac Cardiovasc Surg. 2019;157(4):1696–706.
95. Dzierba AL, Abrams D, Brodie D. Medicating patients during extracorporeal membrane oxygenation: the evidence is building. Crit Care. 2017;21(1):66.
96. Varghese JM, Roberts JA, Lipman J. Antimicrobial pharmacokinetic and pharmacodynamic issues in the critically ill with severe sepsis and septic shock. Crit Care Clin. 2011;27(1):19–34.
97. Ha MA, Sieg AC. Evaluation of altered drug pharmacokinetics in critically ill adults receiving extracorporeal membrane oxygenation. Pharmacotherapy. 2017;37(2):221–35.
98. Wildschut ED, et al. Determinants of drug absorption in different ECMO circuits. Intensive Care Med. 2010;36(12):2109–16.
99. Cheng V, et al. Optimising drug dosing in patients receiving extracorporeal membrane oxygenation. J Thorac Dis. 2018;10(Suppl 5):S629–s641.
100. Shekar K, et al. Sequestration of drugs in the circuit may lead to therapeutic failure during extracorporeal membrane oxygenation. Crit Care. 2012;16(5):R194.
101. Shekar K, et al. Pharmacokinetic changes in patients receiving extracorporeal membrane oxygenation. J Crit Care. 2012;27(6):741.e9–18.
102. Mehta NM, et al. Potential drug sequestration during extracorporeal membrane oxygenation: results from an ex vivo experiment. Intensive Care Med. 2007;33(6):1018–24.
103. Mulla H, et al. Drug disposition during extracorporeal membrane oxygenation (ECMO). Paediatr Perinatal Drug Ther. 2001;4(3):109–20.
104. Preston TJ, et al. In vitro drug adsorption and plasma free hemoglobin levels associated with hollow fiber oxygenators in the extracorporeal life support (ECLS) circuit. J Extra Corpor Technol. 2007;39(4):234.
105. Preston TJ, et al. Modified surface coatings and their effect on drug adsorption within the extracorporeal life support circuit. J Extra Corpor Technol. 2010;42(3):199.
106. Zimmerman KO, et al. Sedative and analgesic pharmacokinetics during pediatric ECMO. J Pediatr Pharmacol Ther. 2020;25(8):675–88.
107. Dreucean D, et al. Approach to sedation and analgesia in COVID-19 patients on venovenous extracorporeal membrane oxygenation. Ann Pharmacother. 2022;56(1):73–82.
108. Rosen DA, Rosen KR, Silvasi DL. In vitro variability in fentanyl absorption by different membrane oxygenators. J Cardiothorac Anesth. 1990;4(3):332–5.

109. Dagan O, et al. Effects of extracorporeal membrane oxygenation on morphine pharmacokinetics in infants. Crit Care Med. 1994;22(7):1099–101.
110. Geiduschek JM, et al. Morphine pharmacokinetics during continuous infusion of morphine sulfate for infants receiving extracorporeal membrane oxygenation. Crit Care Med. 1997;25(2):360–4.
111. Ho ATN, Patolia S, Guervilly C. Neuromuscular blockade in acute respiratory distress syndrome: a systematic review and meta-analysis of randomized controlled trials. J Intensive Care. 2020;8(1):1–11.
112. Combes A, et al. ECMO for severe ARDS: systematic review and individual patient data meta-analysis. Intensive Care Med. 2020;46(11):2048–57.
113. Kressin C, et al. Cisatracurium continuous infusion versus no neuromuscular blockade for acute respiratory distress syndrome on venovenous extracorporeal membrane oxygenation. J Clin Pharmacol. 2021;61(11):1415–20.
114. DeGrado JR, et al. Evaluation of sedatives, analgesics, and neuromuscular blocking agents in adults receiving extracorporeal membrane oxygenation. J Crit Care. 2017;37:1–6.
115. Satyapriya S, Lyaker M, Rozycki A. Sedation, analgesia delirium in the ECMO patient. In: Extracorporeal membrane oxygenation-advances in therapy. Rijeka: IntechOpen; 2016.
116. Roy J, Varin F. Physicochemical properties of neuromuscular blocking agents and their impact on the pharmacokinetic–pharmacodynamic relationship. Br J Anaesth. 2004;93(2):241–8.
117. Kisor DF, Schmith VD. Clinical pharmacokinetics of cisatracurium besilate. Clin Pharmacokinet. 1999;36(1):27–40.
118. Atherton DPL, Hunter JM. Clinical pharmacokinetics of the newer neuromuscular blocking drugs. Clin Pharmacokinet. 1999;36(3):169–89.
119. Ostermann M, Lumlertgul N. Acute kidney injury in ECMO patients. Annu Update Intensive Care Emerg Med. 2021;2021:207–22.
120. Roth C, et al. Liver function predicts survival in patients undergoing extracorporeal membrane oxygenation following cardiovascular surgery. Crit Care. 2016;20(1):1–7.

Chapter 10
Pharmacology and Anticoagulation in ECMO

Kayla A. Lawlor

Normal Hemostasis and ECMO

The human body strives to maintain homeostasis via many regulatory processes and feedback mechanisms, and the ability of the body to maintain endogenous hemostasis and anticoagulation is no exception. Classically, the clotting cascade model of coagulation is described with two major pathways for triggering the blood clotting cascade: (1) the tissue factor pathway or extrinsic pathway activated by trauma and (2) the contact pathway or intrinsic pathway activated by the blood (and factors) making contact with a foreign surface; both of these pathways culminate in the same result known as the final common pathway as demonstrated in Fig. 10.1 [15]. It was previously believed that the intrinsic pathway was not activated in vivo and resulted from contact with a foreign body (hence the contact pathway name). Newer theories on the clotting cascade suggest that these pathways augment each other simultaneously, more specifically that the contact pathway amplifies the tissue factor pathway in three phases of coagulation [4, 15]. Both are mentioned here for completeness, acknowledging that both rely heavily on the chain activation of factors and positive feedback loops to achieve hemostasis, and this complex interdependent network serves to prevent spontaneous thrombosis in healthy humans.

Extracorporeal membrane oxygenation (ECMO) provides direct interference with the body's normal pathways, leading to a state that can be both prothrombotic and coagulopathic. As blood is exposed to a large surface area of foreign, non-human material (the pump, membrane oxygenator, cannula tubing, etc.) continuously during the process of ECMO, proteins from the blood adsorb to all these

K. A. Lawlor (✉)
Department of Anesthesiology, Emory University School of Medicine – Adjunct Clinical Instructor, Atlanta, GA, USA
e-mail: kayla.lawlor@emoryhealthcare.org

157

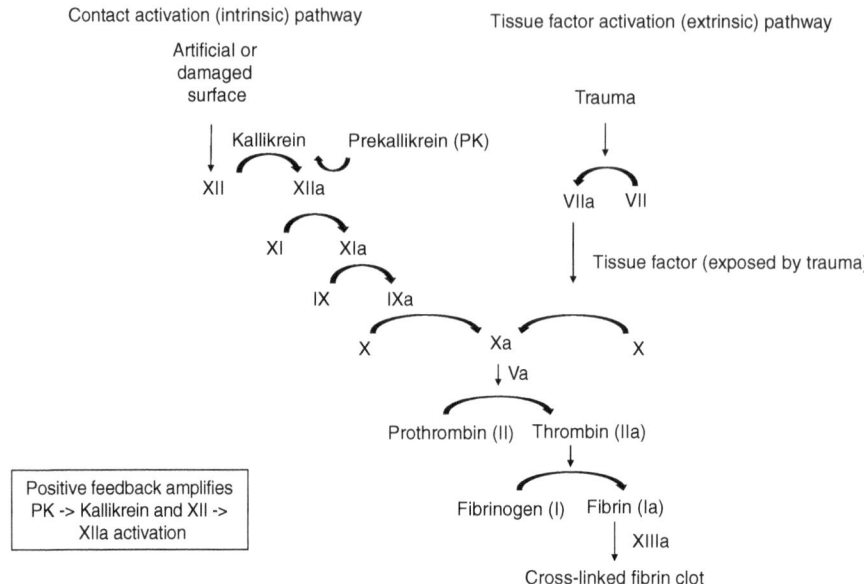

Fig. 10.1 Clotting cascade

ECMO surfaces. Fibrinogen, von Willebrand factor (vWF), and factor XII are all known to adhere to the ECMO foreign body material and activate the intrinsic pathway of the clotting cascade [8]. This results in several notable concurrent processes; firstly, the clotting cascade is now activated on the surface of the ECMO circuit, leading to clots in the cannulas, in the oxygenator, and on the pump itself. Secondly, these clotting factors are being depleted from the patient as they are consumed and accumulate on the ECMO circuit, leaving the patient at a theoretical bleeding risk with the absence of endogenous clotting factors; in fact, one single-center study of 59 patients initiating VV ECMO demonstrated that 100% of patients had vWF deficiency one day after cannulation. These patients also demonstrated functional platelet impairment, which is to be expected due to the role of vWF in platelet aggregation [7]. This highlights the unique need of the ECMO patient in managing anticoagulation as they teeter between a state of prothrombotic intrinsic clotting cascade activation and a state of coagulopathy resulting from consumption of clotting factors and the resulting functional impairment of platelets.

Anticoagulation in ECMO

Anticoagulation in an ECMO patient is a balance of bleeding and clotting risk. Hemorrhage remains the most common complication from ECMO therapy with a reported incidence between 30 and 60% [2] (Thiagarajan 2017), while the known thrombotic risk of ECMO requires the use of anticoagulation in spite of this hemorrhagic concern. As a result of this, the ideal anticoagulant in ECMO patients has many specific criteria. The ideal anticoagulant for ECMO demonstrates a rapid onset and a quick offset and/or with a known reversal agent in case of hemorrhage. This anticoagulant would additionally demonstrate predictable pharmacokinetics not reliant on end organ function to metabolize for the pharmacokinetics in case of multi-system organ failure.

Due to their long duration of action and questionable enteral absorption in the setting of critical illness, all enteral anticoagulants including vitamin K antagonists are not used in patients while they are receiving active ECMO therapy. Likewise, subcutaneous anticoagulation with low molecular weight heparins can experience variable absorption and demonstrate a long half-life, making these agents poor choices as well. Unfractionated heparin (UFH) continuous infusion remains the mainstay of ECMO anticoagulation and the agent recommended by the Extracorporeal Life Support Organization (ELSO) with growing interest in intravenous direct thrombin inhibitors (DTI), namely bivalirudin and argatroban [10]. These agents are discussed in length in the following discussion.

Prior to initiation of any of these agents, baseline coagulation labs, a complete blood count (CBC), and complete metabolic panel (CMP) to establish a patient's current state of organ function and coagulopathy should be attained, including an international normalized ratio (INR), prothrombin time (PT), activated plasma time (aPTT), liver function tests (LFTs), and a serum creatinine to assess renal function. This is important for many reasons. Firstly, patients receiving ECMO are frequently among the highest acuity patient population, such that they require exogenous life support, and this severity of illness often comes with abnormalities in coagulation labs due to sepsis, disseminated intravascular coagulopathy (DIC), and end organ dysfunction. Knowing a patient's baseline derangements can help providers to walk the line between bleeding and clotting for each ECMO patient tailored to the patient's specific needs. Additionally, many patients receive a bolus of anticoagulation (most frequently with heparin but occasionally with a DTI) during ECMO cannulation, and these labs can help detect if the patient is still therapeutically anticoagulated. This can help tailor further guidance for delaying or reducing initial anticoagulation.

Unfractionated Heparin (UFH)

Heparin is one of the oldest pharmaceuticals in widespread clinical use and represents a heterogenous mixture of branched glycosaminoglycans that occur endogenously within humans and are prepared commercially from bovine lung or porcine intestinal mucosa [12]. UFH's mechanism of action primarily relies on binding to antithrombin, a naturally occurring anticoagulant whose anticoagulation ability is potentiated 1000 fold after binding to UFH. Antithrombin was first identified as

Antithrombin 3 or AT by Abdilgaard in 1968, now known as antithrombin (AT) [12]. AT undergoes a conformational change upon binding to heparin which then displays the AT active site of binding for thrombin; this "activated" UFH-AT complex then inactivates free thrombin, resulting in anticoagulation by reducing available thrombin to convert fibrinogen to fibrin [10]. This UFH-AT complex also catalyzes the inactivation of factors IIa, Xa, IXa, and XIIa [6]. Intravenous administration of heparin results in a rapid onset of anticoagulation at therapeutic doses [12].

UFH demonstrates biphasic clearance; first, through the reticuloendothelial system, which is saturable and represents the majority of clearance of heparin at therapeutic doses, and second through slower, non-saturable renal clearance [6]. The half-life of heparin is between 30 and 90 min, and patients with severe renal dysfunction may demonstrate a slightly longer UFH half-life [12].

Dosing of UFH for infusion is weight-based, and the infusion is frequently initiated with an 80 unit/kg bolus followed by a continuous infusion of 12–18 units/kg/h. titrated per therapeutic drug monitoring [6]. It is important to note when initiating a heparin infusion that many patients receive a large heparin bolus during ECMO cannulation, which could render a second bolus with the initiation of the heparin drip to be unnecessary. For titration and adjustment of heparin, many institutions will have a nurse-driven protocol for titration and have a publically available nomogram for heparin titration. There are several therapeutic monitoring options for heparin surveillance: the Activated Clotting Time (ACT), the activated plasma thrombin time (aPTT), and the anti-Xa level are all methods mentioned within the ELSO guidelines and are frequently utilized in practice [10]. Figure 10.2 compares these methods. Other methods that are mentioned as options are the TEG/ROTEM, the plasma dilute thrombin time, and the ecarin clotting time; these methods have limited availability due to cost and so are not as frequently used but are mentioned here to note future directions in UFH monitoring [10].

ACT monitoring assesses the time which is most frequently used with heparin in cardiopulmonary bypass, but this setting targets much higher ACT goals (routinely 400–600 s) than ECMO maintenance anticoagulation (routinely 180–200 s). Complicating this, ACT point of care platforms can vary in their relationship to heparin measured levels, especially at the lower ranges utilized for ECMO [3]. aPTT monitoring similarly demonstrates inter-reagent variability and must be routinely validated in the presence of heparin to maintain reliable titration nomograms. The anti-Xa assay assesses the direct effect of the heparin in its augmentation of AT inhibition of factor Xa, but does not assess the anticoagulation status of the entire blood and so can miss coagulopathies outside of this mechanism. For this reason, many institutions utilize a combination of these methods to assess the anticoagulation status of the patient while on heparin, particularly looking for discordance between a whole blood anticoagulation test and the anti-Xa assay. An example might be if a patient demonstrated a low anti-Xa level at 0.2 IU/mL (with therapeutic routinely being 0.3–0.7 IU/mL) and an aPTT of 65 s (with therapeutic routinely 60–80 s at this institution), the team may decide the patient is anticoagulated appropriately overall and no further up-titration of the heparin may be needed. This is

	Advantages	Disadvantages	Use with DTI	Therapeutic range for anticoagulation
Activated clotting time (ACT)	Whole blood test Point of care test Frequently used in ECMO for LFH Inexpensive Widely available Examines blood response to all factors influencing hemostasis	Affected by clinical factors Measures end point of clotting cascade not specific UFH effect No standardization between ACT devices	Not approved for use with DTI	180–200 sec but varies between ACT platforms Lower than for cardiopulmonary bypass during surgery (which targets 400–800 seconds)
Activated partial thrombin time (aPTT)	Gold standard for UFH outside of ECMO Widely available Point of care test recently available	Plasma test High degree of variability between patients and in single patient Can be influenced by clinical factors and collection techniques No standardization between reagents	Standard for DTI monitoring	40–60 seconds vs 60–80 seconds depending on bleeding risk OR 1.5–2.5 times upper limit normal of test (range depends on reagents at individual lab)
Anti-Xa Assay (heparin activity assay)	Specific to UFH effect on catalysis of AT's inhibition for Factor Xa Less variability with UFH than aPTT	Plasma test No standardization between assay techniques, reagents Chromogenic assay Falsely low anti-Xa results with elevated plasma free hemoglobin, triglycerides, and bilirubin	No, only has monitoring ability for UFH	0.3–0.7 IU/mL Many institutions further separate into low intensity (0.3–0.5 IU/mL) and high intensity (0.5–0.7 IU/mL) to adjust for bleeding risk

Adapted from ELSO 2021 Anticoagulation Guidelines (McMichael 2022)

Fig. 10.2 Anticoagulation monitoring strategies

frequently an interdisciplinary discussion involving the intensivist, the surgeon, the provider (for both ECMO and critical care medicine), the bedside nurse, and the pharmacist to tailor to a patient's specific needs, and goals should be re-assessed regularly for appropriateness as the patient's clinical status evolves. Other factors that may go into the patient's individual titration of anticoagulation include thrombocytopenia, active bleeding or clotting, and liver dysfunction; this highlights again the importance of baseline and routine surveillance of coagulation labs, CBC, and CMP.

Heparin Resistance and Antithrombin (AT) Supplementation

Because heparin is a weight-based medication for initiation that is ultimately titrated to clinical effect on coagulation labs, individual patient dosing needs vary. Additionally, heparin is dependent on endogenous AT to produce its clinical effect of anticoagulation, as it works by potentiation of the anticoagulation effect of AT. Children, specifically infants <1 year of age, naturally display reduced levels of endogenous AT, and adults on ECMO can demonstrate both AT consumption and dilution while on ECMO resulting in lower AT levels. In patients who are receiving high doses of heparin (considered >20 units/kg/min) with persistent subtherapeutic anticoagulation, it is reasonable to consider AT deficiency and check an AT level. Normal plasma AT levels are 15–20 mg/dL [3] but are frequently expressed in lab results as a percentage of normal, with greater than 50% considered as being therapeutic AT levels and a level of 80–100% targeted in AT supplementation [10]. AT concentrate exists with several brands, and each brand has its own equation to calculate dose for supplementation based on weight, current AT level, and goal AT level. An example is here for Thrombate III brand. Repeat doses may be necessary, but frequent AT redosing or persistent heparin resistance may be an indication for switching to a DTI from heparin.

$$\text{Thrombate III dose}(\text{IU}) = \frac{[\text{Desired AT} - \text{current AT level}] \times \text{weight}(\text{kg})}{1.4}$$

Heparin-Induced Thrombocytopenia

Heparin-induced thrombocytopenia, or HIT, is a rare but serious complication of heparin usage, affecting up to 5% of adult patients exposed to heparin [10]. It is an immunological reaction to the complex of heparin and platelet factor 4 (PF4) which occurs due to heparin's negative molecular charge changing the conformation of the PF4 and exposing a neo-epitope which is the HIT antigen, leading to antibody synthesis. These antibodies to the heparin-PF4 complex can cause activation of platelets and subsequent platelet aggregation [9]. This causes thrombocytopenia as a result of platelet consumption and coagulation at both the microvascular and macrovascular level, despite the presence of heparin. This is potentially life-threatening due to the prothrombotic nature of this immune-mediated disease, especially in patients exposed to heparin multiple times and in ECMO patients who are already prothrombotic, this can lead to sudden oxygenator failure and emergent pump exchange [10]. If HIT is suspected, all heparin products must be withdrawn and a direct thrombin inhibitor should be initiated to prevent further thrombus formation and platelet consumption, even in thrombocytopenia.

A screening method called the 4T score can be utilized in patients who have thrombocytopenia in the presence of heparin to assess their risk of HIT. There are four components to the 4T score that assess the patient's thrombocytopenia characteristics and apply them to a HIT traditional diagnosis: degree of thrombocytopenia, timing of thrombocytopenia, the presence of thrombus, and other potential causes of thrombocytopenia. Classically, the degree of thrombocytopenia demonstrated in HIT is >50% decrease with a platelet nadir of 20 or higher; however, many ECMO patients have other mechanical devices (impellas, VADs, etc.) which are also contributing to platelet decrease and so the nadir in an ECMO patient may be lower. The timing for HIT to occur requires antibody formation and so usually the antibody drop starts 5–10 days after initial heparin exposure, although if the patient has been exposed to heparin repeatedly then an immediate drop could be observed. For these confounding reasons in ECMO patients, if HIT is suspected, then diagnostic testing should be sent regardless of 4T score [9].

Many institutions utilize an ELISA assay test for antibodies to the heparin-PF4 to first assess a patient for HIT; these assays are easy to do within institution labs and are highly sensitive to rule out HIT but unspecific and can have false positives. If a HIT ELISA assay is positive, this should prompt a platelet-activation assay or a serotonin release assay (SRA) test to be performed, which is the gold standard for HIT diagnosis. The SRA tests for the serotonin that platelets release when they are activated and aggregate, specifically looking to see serotonin and therefore aggregation in the presence of heparin. A negative SRA result implies no HIT diagnosis, but recent literature shows the risk of false negatives in the setting of platelet inhibiting medications. If a patient demonstrates a negative SRA but had a high HIT ELISA with persistent clinical concern, it is reasonable to consider HIT in the absence of a positive SRA and utilize a DTI. Confirmed HIT requires treatment with a DTI to prevent further coagulation and aggregation of platelets and an allergy of heparin with a reaction of HIT should be documented in the patient's medical record [9], although evidence suggests that a patient's risk of developing HIT returns to normal after the antibodies half-life has passed (3–6 months) [11].

Direct Thrombin Inhibitors

There are two direct thrombin inhibitors that are routinely used in ECMO: argatroban and bivalirudin. Both of these agents work by reversibly binding to thrombin and directly inhibiting thrombin's propagation of fibrinogen to fibrin. Monitoring of these agents can be performed by several tests (see Fig. 10.2) but aPTT is the gold standard for monitoring these agents. The use of one test to assess anticoagulation is considered an advantage of these agents over heparin to many ECMO specialists. Both DTI demonstrate an onset of less than 1 h with initiation of continuous infusion [5, 13]. Argatroban is metabolized hepatically, where bivalirudin demonstrates some renal clearance, thus end organ function can be the deciding factor when choosing between the two agents [10]. However, argatroban demonstrates a prolonged half-life in critical illness and so requires an empiric dose decrease in all ECMO patients with a prolonged duration of action that bivalirudin does not routinely demonstrate. For this reason, some ECMO surgeons feel comfortable with the more predictable pharmacokinetics of bivalirudin in critical illness and therefore ECMO, even in the setting of renal replacement therapy and end organ renal dysfunction, where they may choose to empirically reduce the initial bivalirudin dose to 0.08 mg/kg/h in renal dysfunction or renal replacement therapy compared to a normal bivalirudin initiation dose of 0.15 mg/kg/h [13]. A last factor in the choice between the two agents may be pharmaceutical cost and individual institution purchasing contracts between the manufacturers of these medications. Both DTI medications interact with the INR testing assay, although argatroban does this more dramatically than bivalirudin, with an increase of 2 predicted with argatroban and an increase of 0.5–1 routinely seen with bivalirudin [5, 13]. This is important to remember if a patient is titrating to warfarin and can affect interpretation, again emphasizing the importance of baseline coagulation labs.

Assessment of Bleeding

As discussed, there are a plethora of reasons for an ECMO patient to bleed, including at the cannulation and ECMO sites, the placement of other life sustaining devices, lines, and tubes, procedures, surgical locations, active anticoagulation, consumption of clotting factors, and thrombocytopenia. Bleeding should trigger an interdisciplinary review of the anticoagulation goals and may result in decreasing anticoagulation goals or holding anticoagulation depending on bleed severity and patient hemodynamics. Depending on the need for hemostasis, antifibrinolytics such as aminocaproic acid or tranexamic acid can be used to stop bleeding and promote fibrin clot formation by binding to plasminogen and preventing plasmin formation, thus allowing clot propagation [10]. Both agents can be administered topically at a local site of bleeding on a gauze or systemically as an IV. Aminocaproic acid is dosed as a 5 g intravenous bolus over 1 h followed by a continuous infusion of 1 g per h, due to its short half-life of 2 h [1]. Tranexamic acid has a longer half-life of up to 8 h, and so can be dosed as 1 g IV every 8 h [14].

Conclusion

The balance between bleeding and clotting in a patient receiving ECMO is as delicate as a tightrope and fluctuates frequently as patient condition evolves. Agents such as heparin, argatroban, and bivalirudin can be used to anticoagulate these patients with a variety of monitoring tests to assess the patient's anticoagulation status, while agents such as aminocaproic acid and tranexamic acid can be utilized for hemostasis in a local or systemic level. Ultimately, the patient's individual risk for bleeding and clotting should determine anticoagulation goals, and subjective data should be assessed for safety and efficacy.

References

1. Amicar package insert, FDA. https://www.accessdata.fda.gov/drugsatfda_docs/label/200 4/15197scm036,scf037,scp038,scm039_amicar_lbl.pdf. Accessed 11 Feb 2023.
2. Aubron C, DePuydt J, Belon F, et al. Predictive factors of bleeding events in adults undergoing extracorporeal membrane oxygenation. Ann Intensive Care. 2017;6:97.
3. Chlebowski MM, Baltagi S, Carlson M, et al. Clinical controversies in anticoagulation monitoring and antithrombin supplementation for ECMO. Crit Care. 2020;24:19. https://doi. org/10.1186/s13054-020-2726-9.
4. Colvin BT. Physiology of haemostasis. Vox Sang. 2004;87(S1):S43–6.
5. Dhillon S. Argatroban: a review of its use in the management of heparin-induced thrombocytopenia. Am J Cardiovasc Drugs. 2009;9(4):261–82.
6. Garcia D, et al. Antithrombotic therapy and prevention of thrombosis, 9th Ed: American College of Chest Physicians Evidence-Based Clinical Practice Guidelines. Chest. 2012;141(S2):e24S–43S.
7. Kalbhenn J, et al. Acquired von Willebrand syndrome and impaired platelet function during venovenous extracorporeal membrane oxygenation: rapid onset and fast recovery. J Heart Lung Transplant. 2018;37:985–91.
8. Kumar G, Maskey A. Anticoagulation in ECMO patients: an overview. Indian J Thor Cardiovasc Surg. 2021;37(S2):S241–7.
9. Marchetti M, Zermatten MG, Bertaggia Calderara D, Aliotta A, Alberio L. Heparin-induced thrombocytopenia: a review of new concepts in pathogenesis, diagnosis, and management. J Clin Med. 2021;10(4):683.
10. McMichael A, et al. 2021 ELSO adult and pediatric anticoagulation guidelines. ASAIO J. 2022;2022:303.
11. Selleng S, Haneya A, Hirt S, Selleng K, Schmid C, Greinacher A. Management of anticoagulation in patients with subacute heparin-induced thrombocytopenia scheduled for heart transplantation. Blood. 2008;112:4024–7.
12. Tahir R. A review of unfractionated heparin and it's monitoring. US Pharm. 2007;32(7):HS-26–36.
13. Taylor T, Campbell CT, Kelly B. A review of Bivalirudin for pediatric and adult mechanical circulatory support. Am J Cardiovasc Drugs. 2021;21:395–409.
14. Tranexamic acid package insert, FDA. https://www.accessdata.fda.gov/drugsatfda_docs/ label/2019/212020lbl.pdf. Accessed Feb 11 2023.
15. Versteeg H, et al. New fundamentals in hemostasis. Physiol Rev. 2013;93:327–58.

Chapter 11
Weaning and Decannulation

Ahmed Reda Taha and Ahmed Zaher

Introduction

Intensivists face a challenge when deciding when and how to wean patients from extracorporeal respiratory support. There are no definite criteria for the decision, so the attending physician tends to rely on personal clinical judgment and experience; however, guidelines from scientific societies, hospital protocols, and published case studies may provide some guidelines [1].

Weaning of VV ECMO

Our discussion of the weaning process will include the following points:

(a) When does a patient become ready to wean?
(b) What are the steps involved in weaning?
(c) What are the methods used to manage ventilation during weaning?

As the native lung function improves, extracorporeal support is gradually reduced. Therefore, to determine whether a patient is ready for weaning off ECMO, we recommend a comprehensive assessment of his respiratory function, review predictors of failure (Table 11.1), and monitor variations of the following functional parameters throughout the disease process:

A. R. Taha (✉)
Critical Care Institute, Cleveland Clinic Abu Dhabi, Abu Dhabi, United Arab Emirates

A. Zaher
Oxford Critical Care, Oxford University Hospitals NHS Foundation Trust, Level 1, John Radcliffe Hospital, Oxford, UK

© The Author(s), under exclusive license to Springer Nature Switzerland AG 2024
A. R. Taha et al. (eds.), *ECMO: A Practical Guide to Management*,
https://doi.org/10.1007/978-3-031-59634-6_11

Table 11.1 Predictors for failure to wean from VV-ECMO [2–4]

Parameters	Values of concern	Interpretation
Oxygen saturation	<88%	Late sign of distress
Heart rate	>110	Multifactorial causes
$PaCO_2$	New respiratory acidosis	Late sign of distress
$P_{ET}CO_2/PaCO_2$ ratio	<1	Associated with greater likelihood of failure from VV-ECMO.
Respiratory rate	>35	Late sign of distress
Tidal volume	>8 ml/kg IBW	Depends on respiratory system elastance
Driving pressure	>15 cm H_2O	Evaluates both lung and chest wall
P 0.1	>10 cmH_2O	May be falsely low in patients with respiratory muscle weakness
ΔP_L	>20 cmH_2O	Requires esophageal catheter
Total lung stress (PEEP$_L$ + ΔP_L)	Unknown	Difficult assessment of PEEP$_L$ in patients with abdominal contraction

(a) An increase in native lung oxygen delivery compared to artificial lung oxygen delivery. If the native lung is capable of supporting 50–80% of the total gas exchange, ECMO discontinuation can be considered [5]. Mols et al. reported weaning off ECMO for ARDS when 80% of total oxygen delivery was supplied by the patient's own lung in a large cohort of ARDS patients treated with ECMO.

(b) Improvements on imaging studies, such as improved lung aeration on chest X-rays and resolving B-lines on lung ultrasounds.

(c) An improvement of respiratory mechanics, such as a better static compliance of the respiratory system or a reduction of airway resistance.

(d) Improvement of gas exchange: There is a general consensus that weaning should be considered when the patient meets the following criteria: arterial pO2 and pCO2 are adequate at "moderate ventilator settings" (i.e., FiO2 ≤ 0.6–0.5 and relatively low PEEP), increased CO2 levels in capnometry on rest settings on the ventilator, decrease in sweep gas flow needed to maintain normocarbia, and rapid improvement in SpO2 or PaO2 with increase in FiO2 to 100% (Cilley test) [2]. During the Ciley test, also called the oxygen challenge test, the FiO2 is increased to 100% without any other changes to the ventilator settings. In the event that lung aeration has improved, there should be an immediate increase in oxygen saturation within a few minutes, and a PaO2 of >225 mmHg should be observed at 15 minutes after the increase in FiO2. The Ciley test provides evidence that the patient is ready to advance the ventilator settings and undergo a sweep trial. Nevertheless, a recent single-center study of 253 patients concluded that the oxygen challenge test was not a valid predictor of decannulation readiness from VV-ECMO [2].

Discontinuation Procedure

Discontinuation procedure should begin the moment a patient is placed on extracorporeal life support. This plan should also be discussed daily on patient rounds. The only thing worse than not placing a patient on ECMO soon enough is staying on ECMO longer than is required.

With improving native lung function, extracorporeal support is reduced. Patients with severe hypoxia need high extracorporeal blood flow; once their native lungs recover and contribute significantly to arterial oxygenation, extracorporeal blood flow can gradually be reduced. On the other hand extracorporeal blood flow is low in purely hypercapnic patients, and the magnitude of the assist depends on the sweep gas flow. It is recommended that FiO2 of the sweep gas be reduced before that of the ventilator in the initial phases to avoid oxygen-related toxicity on the native lung. Weaning can be accomplished using a variety of mechanical ventilation strategies. For some patients, ECMO may need to be stopped immediately, such as those who have serious bleeding complications. In these cases, the patient might still be receiving controlled mechanical ventilation while disconnected from ECMO [3]. In most cases, ECMO facilitates the switch from controlled mechanical ventilation to assisted spontaneous breathing, such as pressure-support ventilation or neurally adjusted ventilatory assist. It is evident in this case that there is a complex interplay between respiratory drive, sedation, and ventilatory support; increased sweep gas can be a very effective method of controlling a patient's respiratory drive and may result in a reduction in the dosage of sedatives. By modulating extracorporeal assistance, patients can be weaned off the ventilator more effectively. Furthermore, in some situations, invasive mechanical ventilation should be discontinued such as in the presence of severe immunocompromise; patients on ECMO can be extubated while still on ECMO, and extracorporeal support is only discontinued after they are separated from the ventilator [1].

Lung Recruitment

To initiate weaning process and to have a successful trail off, we should plan a recruitment lung strategy during ECMO support.

It has been reported that acute respiratory distress syndrome (ARDS) patients who undergo venovenous extracorporeal membrane oxygenation (VV-ECMO) and have a high lung recruitment potential have a better prognosis and are less likely to remain on ECMO support and stay in the intensive care unit [6]. Lung recruitability seems to play a significant role in the rapid recovery of patients with severe ARDS, and VV-ECMO remains an advanced form of ECMO support for patients with very severe ARDS. These characteristics might help extracorporeal membrane oxygenation (ECMO) clinicians manage patients with different mechanical ventilation strategies (higher positive end-expiratory pressure [PEEP] or airway pressure release ventilation) earlier in the ECMO support phase and improve the outcome. Using CT for quantitative analysis of lung volumes is an innovative and well-done technique used by Camporota et al. [6] in this small but elegant study. In terms of lung quantitative analysis, CT is the "gold standard technique," but it is time consuming, requires expertise, has a high risk for complications, and requires transfer to the radiology department.

The use of lung sonography can be an alternative method for identifying patients with ARDS who have a potential for lung recruitment and recovery. According to our previous research [7], changes in non-aerated areas in lung-dependent regions of patients with ARDS can be easily assessed by lung sonography with a high correlation between PEEP maneuvers and blood gas analysis. In addition, other researchers have demonstrated that lung sonography can be used to quantify lung aeration in ARDS patients and to guide PEEP strategy [8]. As a noninvasive, radiation-free, easily accessible method, lung sonography remains an attractive method despite its limitations, including its inability to distinguish between hyperinflation and normal lung [9]. It has a relatively good correlation with CT scanning views. Considering the peculiarities of ECMO patients (large atelectatic areas, high risk patients, daily lung assessments), we strongly believe that lung sonography can be applied easily at the bedside in VV-ECMO patients to provide valuable clinical information for both lung

recruitment and lung recovery on a daily basis [10]. In addition to lung sonography, electrical impedance tomography is another emerging technique that can be used in parallel with lung sonography. It has previously been demonstrated that this technique provides dynamic information regarding the distribution of regional wall ventilation in ARDS patients{Vasques, 2019 #18} [11]. There is a need for future studies to test such emerging methodologies in a VV-ECMO population and validate their potential clinical application.

Tracheostomy

A tracheostomy is often considered in patients with severe respiratory failure who undergo venovenous extracorporeal membrane oxygenation (VV-ECMO) because it allows the dosage of sedatives to be reduced, facilitates confirmation of neurological findings, and expedites respiratory rehabilitation. The Extracorporeal Life Support Organization (ELSO) guidelines also state that an early tracheostomy should be considered in patients 5 years of age or older [3]. As compared to delayed tracheostomy, early tracheostomy performed within 7 days of ECMO cannulation may decrease the incidence of VAP during ECMO support in patients with severe ARDS. Additionally, it may shorten the duration of artificial respiration and ECMO, but may not improve the outcome. Further research requires prospective and multicenter studies [12].

When the patient is judged to be ready for weaning based on the above criteria, a trial of discontinuing the extracorporeal support is recommended. ECMO that provides venovenous support does not provide hemodynamic support; as a result, there is no requirement to reduce extracorporeal blood flow during the trial off, unlike venoarterial support.

The trial of venovenous ECMO discontinuation should be performed as follows: *(Review* Fig. 11.1 *to summarize the algorithm)*

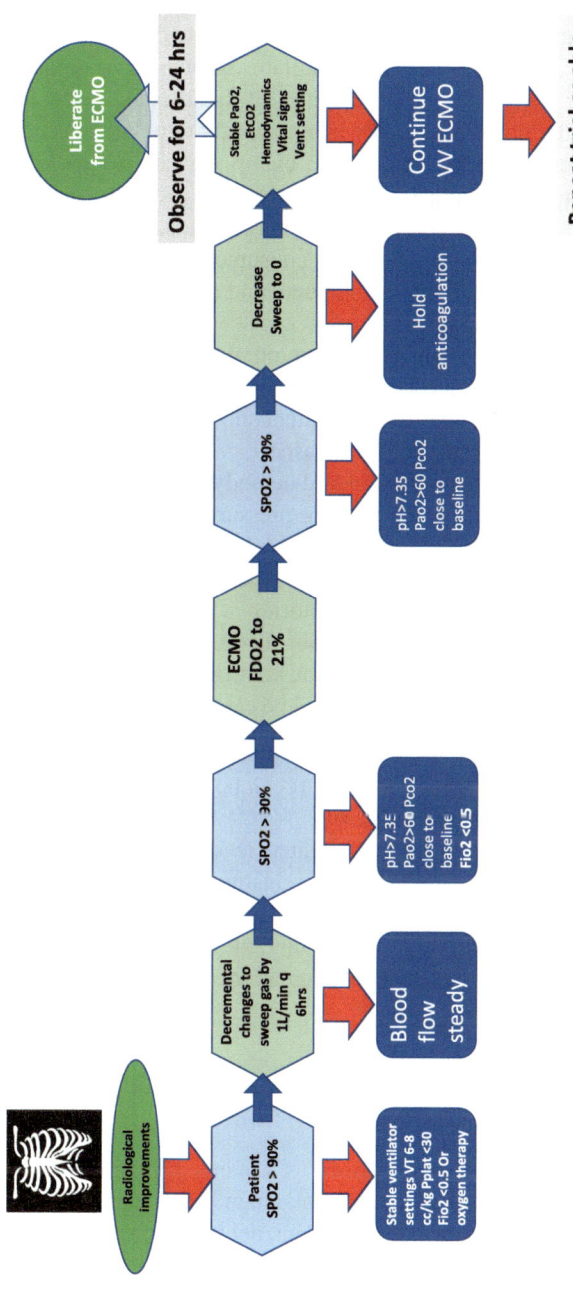

Fig. 11.1 VV-ECMO weaning protocol

1. A patient on controlled mechanical ventilation should be adjusted to a respiration rate, plateau pressure, FiO2, and PEEP that are considered acceptable off ECMO. It may be necessary to adjust the level of inspiratory assist and to adjust the level of sedation if the patient is undergoing assisted spontaneous ventilation (e.g., PSV, ACV, NAVA).• When the ventilator settings have been adjusted, the sweep gas to the oxygenator must be turned off. In order to prevent oxygen from leaking around the flowmeter even when it appears to be off, it is not enough to turn the flowmeter to zero, but also to clamp the gas tubes. Approximately 20 minutes after the sweep gas flow is stopped, the excess oxygen in the extracorporeal circuit will be depleted. Monitoring venous oxygen saturation will reveal when the excess oxygen has been consumed.
2. The extracorporeal blood flow is continued, and no adjustment of heparin dose is required.
3. There are no clear indications on the duration of the trial; some centers suggest a trial off for 1–6 h, but if needed the duration of the trial can be prolonged up to several hours. During this period, the patient should be closely monitored, paying particular attention to the following aspects:
4. Hemodynamic stability: besides standard hemodynamic parameters (heart rate, arterial blood pressure, cardiac filling pressures), continuous monitoring of mixed venous oxygen saturation (if available) is recommended to evaluate the adequacy of oxygen delivery during ECMO discontinuation.
5. Adequacy of gas exchanges (serial monitoring of arterial blood gas analysis).
6. If the patient is on an assisted spontaneous mode of ventilation, respiratory pattern (tidal volume, respiratory rate, minute ventilation), and mechanics (signs of distress, use of accessory muscles) should be carefully assessed [3, 13].

If the patient remains stable during the trial and, most importantly, his ventilatory load is acceptable, the extracorporeal support can be definitively discontinued, and the cannulas removed as described below.

In particularly unstable patients, some centers tend to disconnect the circuit leaving the cannulas in place to allow a prompt reinstitution of the extracorporeal support in case of sudden deterioration of the patient's conditions. Venous cannulas can be left in place for up to 48 hr. to avoid clotting, they should be flushed with a drip of heparinized solution and systemic anticoagulation continued at unchanged dosage.

Decannulation

In most cases, decannulation is performed as a planned bedside procedure after a trial off that shows recovery is adequate to maintain life support through more conventional means. Anticoagulation management, hemostasis, and patient positioning need to be taken into consideration during decannulation. Inotropic and ventilatory therapy is reinstituted if they have been reduced since the trial off. After cannula removal, if necessary, protamine should be administered to correct residual coagulopathy. In addition, a Valsalva maneuver should prevent the venous system from experiencing a significant negative pressure gradient. A surgical approach and repair may be required for arterial cannulae placed. Pressure should be held at the puncture sites for 30 minutes after removal of percutaneously placed venous cannulae.

Direct removal is possible for percutaneously placed cannulas. Some centers recommend turning off heparin 30–60 minutes before decannulation. A purse string suture is applied around the cannulation site before the cannula is removed. As soon as the suture is tightened, local pressure is applied for at least 30 minutes after decannulation. Regularly checking cannulation sites for bleeding or hematomas is recommended.

When removing venous cannulas (especially jugular catheters) in spontaneously breathing patients, there is a potential risk of air aspiration through the catheter's side holes; to avoid this, a Valsalva maneuver on the ventilator should be performed at the time of cannula removal.

After decannulation, we perform a venous Doppler of the lower limbs and of the cannulated vessels to exclude thrombotic events [3].

Some patients may become hypoxemic after decannulation, even after a successful weaning and trial off followed by decannulation. The ventilator settings might need to be optimized in such cases or reintubation if the patient has been extubated. In the case of any patient with ARDS, appropriate diagnostic modalities and appropriate management are required. ECMO support may need to be reconsidered after the family has been informed of the poor prognosis. A study by Mehta [14] concluded that complications are higher during a second course of ECMO support for neonates. Particularly, neurological, infectious, renal, and metabolic complications are more frequent.

Discontinuation for Futility

In the event that the patient's conditions evolve toward permanent and irreversible damage to their brain, lung, and/or heart function, and there is no hope of recovery or organ replacement, the extracorporeal support should be discontinued for futility [15].

Failure to Wean

A successful trial off and weaning may not always be possible. If this occurs, it means we must return to ECMO support. Signs of weaning failure include hypoxia, hypercapnia, respiratory distress, and hemodynamic instability. We need to determine the cause of weaning failure, and we need to consider factors such as patient fatigue, underlying pathology deterioration, sepsis, fluid overload, or inadequate ventilator settings. Diagnostic modalities such as repeat chest X-rays, HRCT chests, or ultrasonography chests should be used to determine the cause. After identifying the cause of failure, we need to correct reversible factors like adequate rest to the patient before weaning, upgrading antibiotics, achieving a negative balance before weaning, and optimizing ventilator settings. During trial off, if only carbon dioxide is retained (PaCO2 > 60 with pH > 7.25) but no hypoxemia occurs, the patient should remain on ECMO or consider arteriovenous carbon dioxide removal (AVCO2 R). Weaning should be attempted again after the underlying cause is corrected [3].

Patients with cardiogenic shock require extracorporeal membrane oxygenation (ECMO), an established strategy for supporting their circulatory system. It is a modality used as a bridge therapy to either implantation of a ventricular assist device or a heart transplantation as a bridge therapy. As ECMO physicians, one of the greatest challenges is to find the best time for venoarterial (VA) ECMO weaning, given that there is no standardized process for weaning VA ECMO. There is limited research on strategies for weaning patients from VA ECMO. Before weaning, we should ensure that the patient is hemodynamically stable and that cardiocirculatory dysfunction is improving. We must also understand that weaning from VA ECMO does not ensure 100% survival. About 35–80% of patients who are weaned off VA ECMO support survive and are discharged [13].

Criteria for Weaning
- Etiology of cardiac dysfunction should be either recoverable or bridging to a therapy.
- Improving cardiocirculatory function, ideally ejection fraction (EF) > 25–30%.
- Hemodynamic stable, with a mean arterial blood pressure (MAP) > 60 mm Hg in the absence of any inotropic support or on minimal inotropic support (inotropic score less than 10).
- A pulsatile arterial waveform should be present for 24 hours.
- SpO2 > 95%.
- ScvO2 > 70%.
- No metabolic derangements.
- Pulmonary function should not be severely impaired.
- Patient must tolerate the weaning trial well.

Predictors of Weaning

During a weaning process, patients should be assessed daily for improvements in clinical status and hemodynamic stability, as well as for improvements on echocardiography. In patients of refractory cardiogenic shock on VA ECMO, various cardiac markers, which indicate myocardial recovery when not on VA ECMO, are usually of no significance, as they are usually elevated in other noncardiac conditions such as sepsis, renal disorders, and multiorgan failure. However, in a study in 2012, Luyt and colleagues observed that prognostic cardiac markers like Troponin I, N-terminal pro-brain natriuretic peptide (NT-proBNP), proadreno-medullin, and copeptin levels are usually elevated in patients with refractory cardiogenic shock on VA ECMO, but their kinetics do not predict any cardiac recovery during the first week of ECMO support. A high lactate level and acidic arterial blood pH are independent risk factors for mortality after ECMO in VA patients. Echocardiography is essential throughout the VA ECMO support process, from initiation to weaning to decannulation. By monitoring the cardiac function, it is possible to predict when ECMO support can be weaned [4].

By evaluating the heart on a daily basis, an intensivist is able to determine its systolic and diastolic function, contractility, valvular abnormalities, and pericardial effusion. Therefore, it explains the causes of weaning failure and assesses the cardiac response to therapeutic interventions. In 2011, Aissaoui et al. identified clinical, hemodynamic, and Doppler echocardiography parameters associated with successfully removing VA ECMO in 51 patients with refractory cardiogenic shock caused by medical (n = 27), postcardiotomy (n = 11), or post-transplantation (n = 5) cardiogenic shock. In all patients weaned off VA ECMO successfully, the LVEF was between 20% and 25%, the aortic velocity-time integral was 10 cm, and the lateral mitral annulus peak systolic velocity was 6 cm/s. As part of a study of postcardiotomy patients, Fiser et al. identified factors that predicted weaning from VA ECMO. The study found that patients with poor EF or elderly patients (>65 years old) were less likely to wean after 48 hours of ECMO [16]. The time survivors spent on ECMO were significantly longer for those with heart transplants.

Echocardiographic findings usually seen during difficult weaning are as follows:

- Regional wall motion abnormalities
- Right ventricular failure
- Left ventricular failure
- Systolic dysfunction
- Diastolic dysfunction
- Mitral regurgitation (postischemic)
- Pericardial tamponade
- Hypovolemia
- Dynamic outflow tract obstruction
- Pulmonary hypertension

Technique for Weaning VA ECMO

In VA ECMO, weaning is not standardized. It is crucial to tailor the weaning strategy based on the initial indication. *(Review* Fig. 11.2 *to summarize the algorithm)*

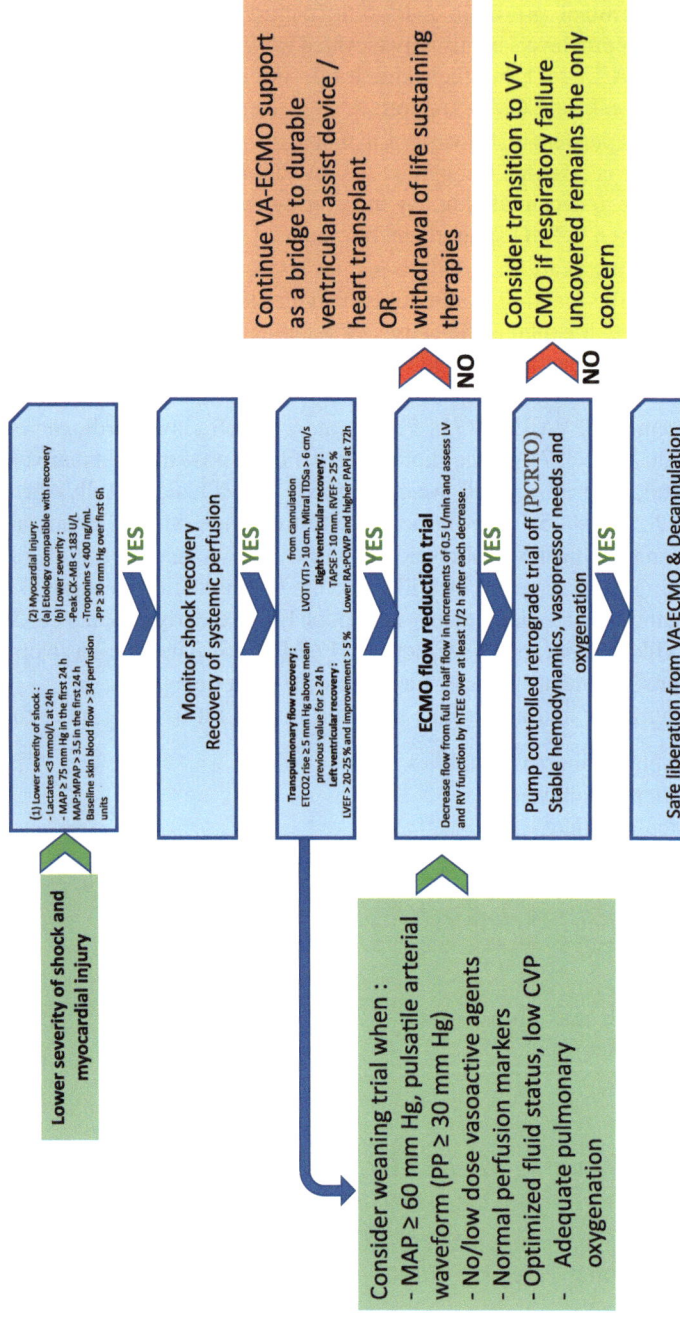

Fig. 11.2 VA ECMO weaning protocol

The primary cause of cardiogenic shock must be resolved before one begins weaning. Myocardial recovery, hemodynamic stability, and the resolution of the primary cause must be achieved before weaning can begin. It is possible to initiate weaning once the patient is hemodynamically stable with minimal or no inotropic support for more than 24 hours and the echocardiogram reveals sufficient myocardial function recovery. The process of weaning involves slowly decreasing the amount of ECMO blood. This results in a reduction in preload and a decrease in afterload, increasing stroke volume and cardiac output. A continuous cardiac function monitoring is performed at every blood flow level of the ECMO pump. A low blood flow is maintained in the ECMO for approximately 40–60 minutes. Ventilatory support is gradually increased based on the increasing pulmonary flow. As a result, the patient is examined for signs of hemodynamic instability, echocardiographic evidence of ventricular insufficiency, and signs of inadequate perfusion, including increased blood lactate levels or a significant fall in ScvO2. It is recommended that full assistance be restored and that the weaning process be restarted after the patient has recovered fully. When the patient remains hemodynamically stable, off inotropes, and LVEF >25–30%, saturation > 95%, and right ventricular pressures are normal, ECMO can be removed. *(Review* Table 11.2 *for Parameters associated with VA ECMO weaning success).*

To avoid clot formation, the patient's heparin infusion is stopped and blood flow is increased to prevent any clots from forming. After ensuring normal coagulation parameters and normal platelet count, the ECMO circuit is clamped and decannulation is performed in the operating room. A blood line and access cannula should be periodically unclamped to avoid stagnation during the trial, according to the Extracorporeal Life Support Organization (ELSO). Some institutes administer levosimendan at 0.1 g/kg/min to improve both systolic and diastolic function, and the activated partial thromboplastin time should be 1.5 to 2.5 times the normal value. Patients on ECMO may be able to survive longer with an intra-aortic balloon pump. According to Petroni et al. [17], intra-aortic balloon pumps restored pulsatility and reduced left ventricular afterload in patients receiving VA ECMO and were associated with smaller left ventricular dimensions and lower pulmonary artery pressure. The value of intra-aortic balloon pumps during VA ECMO weaning has not been evaluated.

Failure to Wean

In case VA -ECMO patients cannot be weaned off, it becomes imperative to identify patients who are suitable for long-term support or transplantation immediately. It is possible to consider mechanical assist devices as either a bridge therapy to transplantation or a destination therapy.

Table 11.2 Parameters associated with VA ECMO weaning success [4]

Parameters	Significance	Advantages	Disadvantages
EtCO$_2$	Higher values at 24 h in weaned patients Rapid rise in EtCO2 preceded changes in hemodynamic monitoring and cardiac index Increase of $\geq$ 5 mmHg above previous mean values during two consecutive 12-h periods associated with weaning and preceded native cardiac output recovery	- Noninvasive alternative to thermodilution cardiac catheter	- Elimination of CO$_2$ may depend on pulmonary dead-space, which is increased after CPR, thus reducing ETCO2 level - May vary with change in ventilator settings
LVEF	Greater increase (>5%) in the first 48 h and significant improvement from cannulation to weaning associated with weaning LVEF > 20–25% reported before attempting weaning trial.	- Direct marker of systolic function;	- Load-dependent - Absolute value at weaning inconsistently predicted weaning success
LVOT VTI	Improvement from cannulation to weaning, values above 8.5 cm at weaning associated with success Threshold of 10 cm reported before attempting weaning trials	- Direct marker of systolic function	- Load-dependent
TDI	Mitral systolic velocities (Sa) higher in weaned patients both at maximal and minimal (>6 cm/s) VA ECMO flow Any improvement in lateral mitral e' velocity and/or > 10% improvement in tricuspid annular S' velocity during flow reduction trial is an independent predictor of weaning success	- Load-independent, making it useful to guide the weaning process - Better predictive performance than conventional parameters for weaning success (interobserver variability)	- Angle-dependent for valid measurement
TAPSE	Higher at full flow (15 mm) in successfully weaned patients		- Limited data - Angle dependency

| RVEF | 3D derived RVEF > 24.6% at first intent of decannulation associated with weaning. Higher RVEF in patients without ventricular interdependence during weaning trial | - Direct marker of systolic function | - Load-dependent
- 3D echo is time consuming and requires offline analysis without immediate assessment
- Two-dimensional measurement less reliable |
| Ventricular interdependence (VI) | Absence of VI (Dep-) on the last day before weaning predicted successful weaning | (A) Highlight ventricular response to load variation | |

ETCO2 Partial pressure of CO_2 in the gas mixture at the end of exhaled breath.

Under constant ventilator settings, its main determinant is transpulmonary flow from the native heart

LVEF Relation between the amount of blood expelled during each cardiac cycle relative to the size of the ventricle.

Velocity-time integral (*VTI*) of a pulsed wave Doppler in the left ventricular outflow tract (LVOT) is directly proportional to the stroke volume of the native heart

Tissue Doppler velocity imaging (*TDI*) is a signal which correlates with myocardial motion. TDI is placed on mitral/tricuspid annulus to evaluate longitudinal systolic function

Tricuspid Annular Plane Systolic Excursion (*TAPSE*) is an M-mode derived marker of longitudinal right ventricular function

RVEF Relation between the amount of blood expelled during each cardiac cycle relative to the size of the ventricle.

Ventricular Interdependence. Phenomenon whereby the function of one ventricle is altered by changes in the filling of the other ventricle.

Post Decannulation

As patients continue to recover, they are focused on further healing, rehabilitation, and preventing further complications. The patient's dyspnea may deteriorate. Perform appropriate diagnostic studies, support respiratory functions with a ventilator, and consider differential diagnosis for worsening conditions (fluid overload, thromboembolism). Systemic inflammatory response syndrome (SIRS) occurs frequently following the decannulation of an ECMO machine. According to Thanappan K et al., "SIRS phenomenon" refers to the presence of 2 out of 3 of the following criteria following ECMO decannulation—fever (temperature > 101.5 °F), leukocytosis [white blood cells (WBCs) > 12,000, or 25% increase from predecannulation baseline] and an increase in vasopressors as compared to predecannulation. We did not use other diagnostic criteria for SIRS, such as increases in heart rate or respiratory rate, as these might depend on the use of inotropes, degree of sedation, and ventilator settings. As early as day one of ECMO decannulation, patients could experience the SIRS phenomenon. It could last almost a week regardless of infection if patients developed SIRS after decannulation. Until culture results are available, patients with SIRS who suspect an infection should be treated aggressively with broad-spectrum antibiotics. Since it is difficult to distinguish between infection and SIRS, empiric antibiotics have been recommended. Whenever a patient is decannulated after 48 hours of ECMO, we administer a bolus dose of vancomycin. In order to optimize hospital outcomes following ECMO decannulation, SIRS must be treated as an infection until proven otherwise [18].

Cessation of Support in Setting of End of Life Care

The majority of patients who are treated with ECMO will be able to wean or bridge to a transplant successfully. Others, however, are unable to recover. As the primary disease may not resolve, there may be contraindications to transplant, and ECMO complications (particularly intracranial hemorrhage) may alter the course of the illness; or critical illness can transform a desperate situation into a downward spiral that cannot be reversed. Despite weeks, even months, of ECMO support, some patients will recover. Therefore, decisions to terminate support should not be taken lightly [19].

Determining the futility of continued critical care is controversial and extremely complex [19, 20], perhaps even more so in the context of patients requiring ECLS [15, 21]. The process of making difficult decisions is facilitated when clear goals are established before ECMO is initiated and these goals are revisited on a regular basis. A clear statement of the purpose of ECMO should be provided to the healthcare team as well as the patient (or surrogate) upon its inception. In the case of ECMO support used as a bridge to transplantation, it is imperative to assess candidacy realistically and ensure that there are no contraindications to transplantation which may strand the patient on a "bridge to nowhere." A more difficult task is defining goals for patients undergoing a bridge to recovery, since the process can be long and hard to predict accurately, and the course may be punctuated with periods of downturn that make survival seem unlikely. In addition to addressing the patient's status, progress toward the goals (or regression), and prognosis, the ECLS team should meet with the patient regularly. In the case of patients who are unlikely to survive, the concept of a time-limited trial (in which explicit metrics and a clear schedule are outlined) [22] can be very beneficial to them and their families.

It is ethically acceptable to withdraw ECLS when the caregivers and the patient agree that it cannot achieve its goals and should be withdrawn. Considering this situation, we recommend focusing on comfort and eliminating all unnecessary interventions in the intensive care unit. The fact that ECLS is not used as a destination therapy leads to the conclusion that terminating it is similar to withdrawing other life-sustaining treatments. Even so, since withdrawal generally leads to immediate death, some discomfort is to be expected, particularly in the care of conscious patients. [23].

As soon as a decision to discontinue ECMO has been made for a patient who is expected to die, the decision should be communicated to all parties involved, including primary caregivers, consultants, referring physicians, nurses, perfusionists, therapists, and other stakeholders. It may be beneficial to involve palliative care specialists and spiritual care services [23]. The patient's comfort should be attained by administering analgesics and sedatives as necessary and anticipating that withdrawal of VV-ECMO may cause or exacerbate dyspnea. As a result, we turn off the sweep gas, preventing further gas exchange in the membrane. The termination of ECMO support, assuming it was life-sustaining, will result in death. VA ECLS patients may experience reduced circuit blood flow after vasoactive drug infusions are discontinued. Keeping the patient comfortable is important in order to prevent worsening dyspnea or any other perceived discomfort [23].

Post-ECMO Follow-up (in Hospital and Post-Discharge)

In order to be able to leave the hospital after successful ECMO weaning and awakening, survivors require complex care, including physical and cognitive rehabilitation, nutritional support, and re-socialization. However, the story does not end at discharge. There is a need to provide routine outpatient visits to ECPR survivors, since there is a chance that they will have ongoing health conditions (the so-called vulnerable period), and that all the efforts and financial resources spent on the acute care may be undermined by inadequate post-discharge care. According to a single-center observational study, ECMO survivors have significantly lower quality of life than controls at 12 months after surgery [24]. Despite this, there is a lack of data regarding the long-term risk of cardiovascular events and survival. It is important that psychological, spiritual, or palliative support is available on an ambulatory basis or even through home care.

References

1. Tonna JE, et al. Management of adult patients supported with venovenous extracorporeal membrane oxygenation (VV ECMO): guideline from the extracorporeal life support organization (ELSO). ASAIO J. 2021;67(6):601–10.
2. Hartley EL, et al. Prediction of readiness to decannulation from venovenous extracorporeal membrane oxygenation. Perfusion. 2020;35(1_suppl):57–64.
3. MacLaren G, et al. Extracorporeal life support: the ELSO red book 6th edition. Extracorporeal Life Support Organization - USA; 2022.
4. Aissaoui N, et al. Predictors of successful extracorporeal membrane oxygenation (ECMO) weaning after assistance for refractory cardiogenic shock. Intensive Care Med. 2011;37(11):1738–45.
5. Mols G, et al. Extracorporeal membrane oxygenation: a ten-year experience. Am J Surg. 2000;180(2):144–54.
6. Camporota L, et al. Lung recruitability in severe acute respiratory distress syndrome requiring extracorporeal membrane oxygenation. Crit Care Med. 2019;47(9):1177–83.
7. Stefanidis K, et al. Lung sonography and recruitment in patients with early acute respiratory distress syndrome: a pilot study. Crit Care. 2011;15(4):R185.
8. Bouhemad B, et al. Bedside ultrasound assessment of positive end-expiratory pressure-induced lung recruitment. Am J Respir Crit Care Med. 2011;183(3):341–7.
9. Stefanidis K, et al. Sonographic lobe localization of alveolar-interstitial syndrome in the critically ill. Crit Care Res Pract. 2012;2012:179719.
10. Vasques F, et al. How I wean patients from veno-venous extra-corporeal membrane oxygenation. Crit Care. 2019;23(1):316.
11. Vasques F, et al. Monitoring of regional lung ventilation using electrical impedance tomography. Minerva Anestesiol. 2019;85(11):1231–41.
12. Zhang Z, et al. Early tracheostomy for ARDS patients supported by venovenous extracorporeal membrane oxygenation is associated with a decreased incidence of ventilator-associated pneumonia, duration of extracorporeal membrane oxygenation and mechanical ventilation: experience from a single-center retrospective cohort. Research Square. Extracorporeal Life Support Organization - USA; 2021.
13. Schmidt GA, SpringerLink. Extracorporeal life support for adults. 1st 2016 ed, Respiratory medicine. New York/Imprint: Springer/Humana; 2016.
14. Mehta T, Sallehuddin A, John J. The journey of pediatric ECMO. Qatar Med J. 2017:2017(1 – Extracorporeal Life Support Organisation of the South and West Asia chapter 2017 conference proceedings).
15. Rosenberg AA, et al. Prolonged duration ECMO for ARDS: futility, native lung recovery, or transplantation? ASAIO J. 2013;59(6):642–50.
16. Fiser SM, et al. When to discontinue extracorporeal membrane oxygenation for postcardiotomy support. Ann Thorac Surg. 2001;71(1):210–4.
17. Petroni T, et al. Intra-aortic balloon pump effects on macrocirculation and microcirculation in cardiogenic shock patients supported by venoarterial extracorporeal membrane oxygenation*. Crit Care Med. 2014;42(9):2075–82.
18. Thangappan K, et al. Systemic inflammatory response syndrome (SIRS) after extracorporeal membrane oxygenation (ECMO): incidence, risks and survivals. Heart Lung. 2016;45(5):449–53.
19. Siegel MD. End-of-life decision making in the ICU. Clin Chest Med. 2009;30(1):181–94. x
20. Luce JM. A history of resolving conflicts over end-of-life care in intensive care units in the United States. Crit Care Med. 2010;38(8):1623–9.
21. Abrams DC, et al. Ethical dilemmas encountered with the use of extracorporeal membrane oxygenation in adults. Chest. 2014;145(4):876–82.
22. Schenker Y, et al. Discussion of treatment trials in intensive care. J Crit Care. 2013;28(5):862–9.
23. Cook D, Rocker G. Dying with dignity in the intensive care unit. N Engl J Med. 2014;370(26):2506–14.
24. Spangenberg T, et al. Health related quality of life after extracorporeal cardiopulmonary resuscitation in refractory cardiac arrest. Resuscitation. 2018;127:73–8.

Index

© The Editor(s) (if applicable) and The Author(s), under exclusive license to
Springer Nature Switzerland AG 2024
A. R. Taha et al. (eds.), *ECMO: A Practical Guide to Management*,
https://doi.org/10.1007/978-3-031-59634-6

GPSR Compliance

The European Union's (EU) General Product Safety Regulation (GPSR) is a set of rules that requires consumer products to be safe and our obligations to ensure this.

If you have any concerns about our products, you can contact us on ProductSafety@springernature.com

In case Publisher is established outside the EU, the EU authorized representative is:

Springer Nature Customer Service Center GmbH
Europaplatz 3
69115 Heidelberg, Germany

Batch number: 10091867

Printed by Printforce, the Netherlands